# GET FIT AT HOME:

## HOME EXERCISES FOR YOU.

### GANIHU ONYEBUASHI

# CONTENTS

# INTRODUCTION

We're often told that the key to living a healthy lifestyle is to incorporate physical activity in our everyday lives, but sometimes it's difficult for us to find the time or motivation to go out and do these activities. And while staying in shape is an integral part of a healthy lifestyle, it can be even more important as we age. The benefits of a healthy lifestyle are several. It can help us to maintain good health and live for an extended period of time. If we don't do it, we may become more vulnerable to chronic diseases and other illnesses that shorten the amount of time we have with our loved ones.

Many studies show that regular exercise can decrease the risk of heart disease, stroke, diabetes, high blood pressure and osteoporosis among many others. Regular exercise also helps us build strength and muscle mass—both factors which could potentially increase our longevity. Physical activity also helps relieve stress, lowers our risk of depression and can help us to get a good night's sleep.

In reality most of us have a hard time finding the time to exercise regularly. We may not always feel like it, or it may be cold or rainy out and we don't want to run outdoors. And if we feel like our schedule is already packed, it can be hard to see how to fit it all in. This is especially true for all of us who work full-time jobs and have busy family lives.

There are various exercises that you can do in your own home on your own time, while you are watching television or just talking on the phone. These home exercises can be used at any time of the day, or on days when you don't feel like exercising. After all, even if you're not feeling like exercising, many of these exercises can do wonders for your body.

There's a lot of ways to stay in shape, from regular cardio workouts to weight training. But there is no one right way—it is simply up to the individual to find the kind of physical activity that will work best for them. Whatever form of exercise it may be, it's important we choose an activity we enjoy so that we have the motivation needed to stick with it and reap all its benefits.

In this book, we've provided several different home exercises that you can incorporate into your daily routine to help you get fit at home. Try a few of these exercises when you're beginning your new workout routine to help you get comfortable with the activity. It's also a good idea to consult your doctor before starting any exercise program to ensure there are no contraindications or other issues that may hinder your efforts.

It's really important and you must listen to your body and be patient. Don't be discouraged if some of these exercises cause some mild discomfort. By steadily increasing the intensity of your workouts, you'll be able to work through the soreness and be rewarded with both a healthy body and a healthy mind.

But exercising can be hard sometimes—even if we know that it's good for us. For some people, getting started of a good workout routine is the most challenging part. I have some tips that can help you get started. Besides, if you need encouragement, there are also tips that will help you to feel more motivated to exercise.

Motivation is a great way to help you stick to your exercise routine, and this book will offer you plenty of ideas on how to stay motivated as you build your fitness level. If you will learn how to recognize the signs and symptoms of low energy or fatigue, you can gain the motivation you need to stay active. It may not feel easy at first, but once you start seeing some results it will motivate you to continue on with your journey.

There are many different ways to stay motivated, which is why each exercise is accompanied by a simple yet effective trick that will serve as a reminder for you to make time in your schedule for exercise. It is really important to try and stay consistent with your exercise routine.

Introducing a challenging workout routine can also help you to stay motivated. By introducing challenging workouts you will be increasing your productivity and staying active in a healthy way. It is important to remember that whenever you are starting out, you should start slowly and give yourself time to warm up and cool down properly. If you will learn how to listen to your body, you will be able to push yourself at the right intensity level so that your body remains challenged while avoiding injury.

By providing you with several different home exercises, you will be giving yourself plenty of options for staying active. It is important that you keep your body guessing so that it is constantly adapting to new challenges. By switching up your exercise routine and challenging your body to adapt, you will be able to burn off more calories and ultimately increase endurance levels and metabolism.

As we grow older, our body becomes more sensitive to certain activities and it is important that we take it easy when we are starting out. By knowing the signs and symptoms of overdoing it, you can become more aware of what your body needs. By staying aware and being sensitive to your body, you will be able to remain active in a healthy way.

# BENEFITS OF HOME EXERCISES

Being healthy is vital to living a long and happy life. Home exercises are an option for people who find traditional workouts boring or uncomfortable. What's more, there is no need to go far just for a workout. With home fitness equipment, you can get in your workout anywhere and anytime.

Home exercises are very effective for people who don't have enough time or money to go to the gym. They are a very good alternative that not only helps people stay in shape without spending any money but also saves them money. Home exercises will give people a chance to get fit without spending anything.

There are various forms of home exercises. They include simple bench presses, squats and even cable exercises. These exercises help people lose fat at home by burning calories and building muscles as well as toning their bodies.

Home exercises are good for people of all ages. Whether you want to lose weight, tone up or get stronger, these exercises will definitely help you achieve the goals that you have in mind. Home exercises are safe and a lot easier to perform when compared with traditional workouts done in gyms or fitness centers.

Home exercises are convenient for people who have back problems as they take away the pressure of standing up and lifting heavy weights. You can even get into the workout with other family members or friends to keep you motivated. You can even modify the exercises to suit your needs.

At home exercises you can do your workouts at any time while doing other daily tasks like cleaning your house, doing laundry, cooking food or even watching TV.

Home exercise equipment will help you stay fit and healthy without having to go to gyms and spend money on expensive membership fees or getting into a long-term contract with a gym. You can get everything that you need in your home for a low price. You can even modify and change exercises to suit your needs.

One thing that most people do not know is that you can burn more calories by doing less exercises. The body cannot only tolerate a certain number of repetitions per exercise but also the number of sets or repetitions in one set. With home exercises, you are able to perform the exercise routine at your own pace and with as many or as few reps as you want without any kind of pressure or commitment.

Home exercise is a great way to bond with the family while having fun at the same time. This way, everyone gets a good workout without feeling uncomfortable or out of shape. You will definitely have more energy and feel healthier after your workout sessions.

Home exercises are not only for fitness lovers. In fact, people in their fifties and sixties can benefit from these exercises especially those who live alone. This is because, with home exercises, you have a way to stay fit even when you are alone and need to stay in shape simply for your own health.

## DETERMINE WHICH EXERCISES ARE BEST FOR YOU

Exercise is a great way for us to stay healthy and maintain a good weight. While people find that exercise can be difficult and time consuming, it doesn't have to be this way because there are many exercises you can do from the comfort of your home.

The first thing that you should do when considering home exercises is consider which are best for you. Certain exercises may not be the best match for you depending on your current situation and health. For example, if you have existing injuries or medical conditions, working with a physician to determine what exercises would be best for you is important. Next, work out your muscles in different ways. For example, some people find that crunches are not the best exercise for them because they feel like their stomach is being squeezed. This may mean that an exercise such as sit-ups would be a better choice because they do not involve the stomach muscles being worked out. When you work your muscles in different ways, it can help you get used to them and provide more muscle definition over time.

To determine how often you should exercise, you should choose an exercise that you can do multiple times per day. For example, if you only have time to do crunches, that may mean doing them once a day or less depending on how long it takes to do the exercises. While this may be fine for some people, working out your muscles more often will ensure that they are getting stronger and receiving more benefits in the long run. When deciding how often you should work out, consider how tired you are the day after exercising. If you are tired, it may be a good idea to do the same exercise multiple times in one day. For example, if you want to work out your thighs on Monday and Tuesday, it may be a good idea to do leg exercises on Monday and arms exercises on Tuesday.

When deciding on the kind of home exercises you want to do, it is also a good idea for you to take into account how much time and energy each exercise will take. You have to make sure that you can fit your home exercises into your schedule. Home exercise programs can be completed at any time of day so if you are busy you don't have to wait for a specific time. With online programs, you don't have to worry about what time of day you want to work out because the program can be started at any time.

Lastly, you must ensure that you determine what exercises are best for you by doing research. You could try to find exercise books or online programs that will give you a description of different exercises. Alternatively, ask friends and family members for advice about their favorite exercises. If they can give recommendations they may have used the same workout before so they know which exercises work best for them.

## HOW TO PLAN YOUR HOME EXERCISES

Planning your home exercises is essential for making sure that they are effective and for providing you with the right amount of space to work. Determine which exercise you want to do, and then plan your movements in a way that will allow you to complete the exercise. It is also a good idea to ensure that you have enough space to position yourself, so be sure to use the measurements suggested in each exercise.

### Planning exercise routine

Planning your exercise routine is essential for making sure that you are doing the right exercises for your body at the right time. It is best to do home exercises on an empty stomach as hunger can increase your heart rate and make you feel weak or irritable, so why not do it in the morning as soon as you wake up (assuming you don't have any early meetings or appointments of course). If you have scheduled a work out for the day, but aren't sure if you are feeling up for it, then don't do it or plan for a second session later in the day. You want to set up your home exercises so that you can get up and do them with minimal effort in the morning and throughout the day.

### A few pointers for home exercises

Some home exercises require different equipment, so make sure that you know what you will need before setting up your workout. If not, then it would be better to switch the exercise than to have to get up and find a piece of equipment or even wait until you go out later in the day. Some home exercises are more effective if done immediately after eating, they can also be easier to do without any distractions. While it is always great to have something to look forward to, your workout should not be the last thing that you do before going out in the evening. In order to get a good workout and still save time for other things during the day, try doing home exercises on an empty stomach and before going out at night.

### Putting together a home exercise regime

When thinking about doing some exercises at home, prioritize their effectiveness over their convenience. If you're going to do the same exercises every day, then it won't be as effective. You always want to start your day with an exercise that gets your heart rate up, but not so much that you are feeling tired the next day. You should also change your routine up so that you don't get bored.

In order to plan and keep track of your workout regime, make a home exercise logbook.

### Planning your home exercises

To put together a home exercise plan, start by breaking down what you want to achieve. If you've been sitting for the past few months and want to get fit, then it is important to know what your goals are and how far you really can go. If you want to be healthy for the long term, then you need to target very specific goals. The more you create a detailed plan is, the better. How much weight do you want to lose? How many inches? What are your health aims? Determining what you plan on achieving is an important part of setting up your home workout regime.

*Exercise goals should be clearly defined*

It is very important to define what you are after and what you want to achieve. If you have been inactive for the past three years, it is not realistic that you are going to look like a fitness model or perform at the same level as a professional athlete, but by knowing what your goals are, you can set yourself up for success in the long-term.

If you really don't know where to start, then it would be better to start small than not start at all. If you've been sitting for a while, start by doing at least 20 minutes of exercise a day, 5 days a week. If this is too much for your body to handle, then start by doing the most effective exercises for your body type and work up from there.

*Planning your home exercises should be easy*

If you are not really sure on how to get started, then it would be better to try something small and manageable than to make a plan that requires several pieces of equipment or an extra person around to help you out. Just by knowing what is possible, you can set yourself up for success in the long term.

2

# WORKOUTS FOR BEGINNERS

A workout for beginners is a general term that describes activities designed to help individuals become fit or more flexible by doing exercises they have never tried before. These workouts are not designed as a long-term fitness program but only to introduce people to the health benefits of exercise and the possibilities of healthier living.

Home exercises can be done at any time, and can be done anywhere you have a comfortable chair or a small floor space.

As a beginner is it easy to start with these exercises. The key to all workouts is stretching and warming up but don't tire yourself out too much as this will prevent you from doing longer workouts, which are better for burning calories.

Start with these easy exercises, and as you become fit, you can add more moves to your workout.

When exercising, aim for a state of fatigue in which you do not feel like you can do more repetitions of an exercise. Then take a short break before repeating the exercise.

Home workouts are simple, affordable and most injury-free. There is no such special skills or equipment required. Go through each exercise routine until your muscles feel tired, then take a break, have a snack and repeat the routine again for about 30 minutes.

A good home workout is one that does not require a lot of time. It's easy to get bored quickly if you're working out for too long. As a beginner, one of the best things you can do is stop pushing yourself too far or trying to do too much, too soon.

You don't always need to buy any equipment for home workout exercises. All you need is the space you will use for the workout and enough time for stretching and other warm-up exercises that prepare your body for exercise.

Exercises for beginners can be fun and you can develop a healthy lifestyle that will keep you fit, strong and in good shape for years to come. Make sure your first workout is not too intense, but do not do push-ups or forms of exercise where you stress your joints or muscles beyond their capability.

## HOME EXERCISES FOR BEGINNERS

There's a reason people say that the best exercise is the one you don't have to leave your home for, it lets you stay in bed and still get fit.

Luckily, there are plenty of exercises for beginners that can be done right from your computer chair or couch at home and this list has a variety of choices.

**#1: Burpees:** The Burpee is a full-body exercise that can help tone and strengthen your arms, abs, chest, and legs. To perform, stand with your feet shoulder-width apart and hands on your hips. Bend down and place your hands on the floor in front of you. Kick both feet back towards your bum, then jump up to return to standing position with hands-on hips again. Repeat as many times as you like.

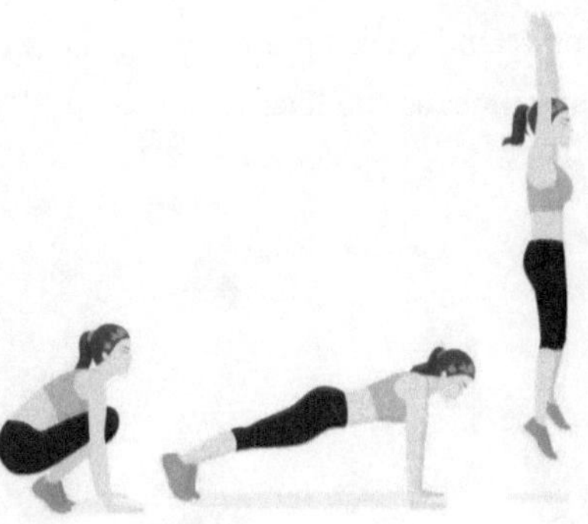

**#2: The Squat:** Squat is one of the best traditional construction exercises for all muscle groups. To do it, begin by standing with your weight on your heels and your arms at your side. Then, slowly bend down and touch the floor with your fingers like you're sitting in a chair. This is the starting position. Return to the starting position, pushing up the floor with both legs at once. Repeat as many times as you like.

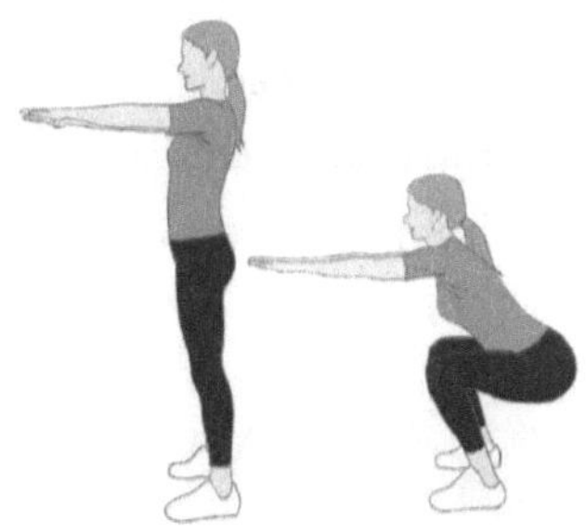

**#3: Kettlebell Swing:** The kettlebell swing is a fantastic exercise for beginners because it's very simple to perform and can be done with just one arm. To do this, grab a kettlebell by the handle and place it on the floor in front of you. Curl up, hinging at the hips so that your back and shoulders are as straight as possible. As you lower your hips towards the floor, slowly bend your knees at the same time. Once your hips are at the bottom of the swing, stand back up and swing the weight back up to finish. Repeat as many times as you like.

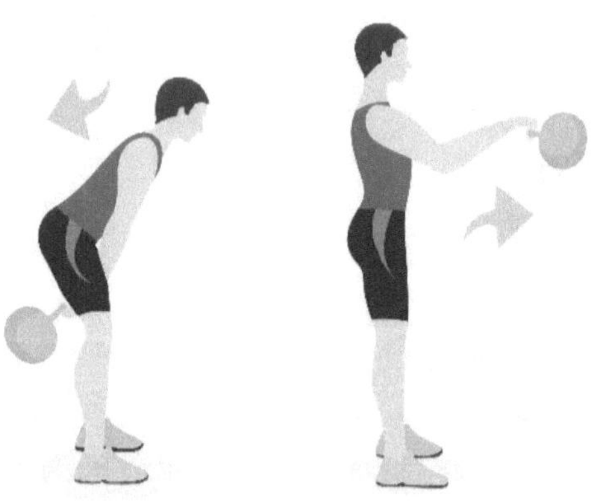

**#4: Push-Up:** The push-up is an excellent exercise for strengthening your arms and chest while toning and shaping your upper body. To do a push-up, you'll need a place to lay down. That place should be next to two bricks or two boxes stacked on top of each other. First, get on the floor with your hands and feet about hip-width apart. Next, lower yourself, chest down, to the floor. Then push yourself back up to a standing position by straightening your arms at the elbows. Repeat as many times as you like.

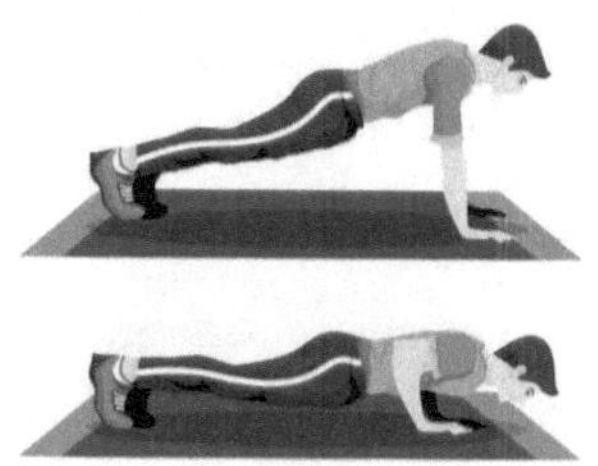

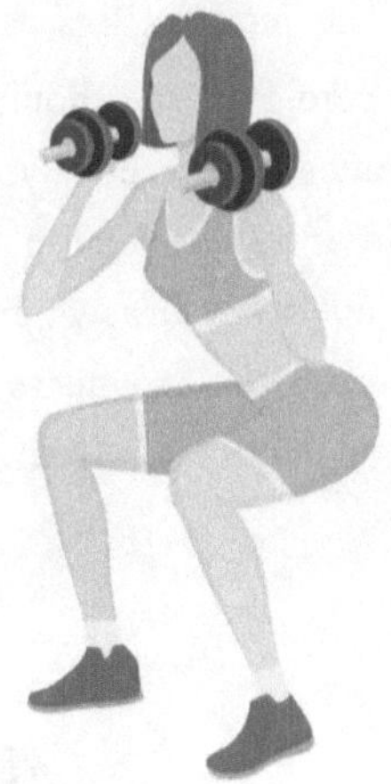

**#5: Squats with Weight:** The squat is a great exercise for anyone of any fitness level and is considered one of the keystone exercises of all time. It can be performed and you can use a barbell or dumbbells in your home. To do this, grab two dumbbells and hold them at your sides as you stand up straight. Begin by slowly standing up as tall as possible, making sure to keep your back and legs straight. Then, bend at the knees so that you're sitting on a chair with your thighs parallel to the floor. Return to standing by pushing through the floor with both legs at once. Repeat as many times as you like.

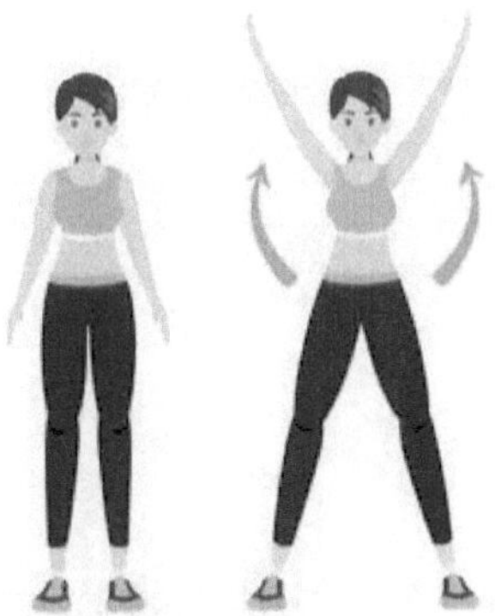

shutterstock.com · 1457642288

**#6: Jumping Jacks:** The jumping jack is an excellent exercise for gaining strength in your core, legs, and shoulders. To execute this, stand with your feet together and arms up above your head with hands touching. Spread your legs apart as wide as you can go so that they're parallel to the ground. Then jump up in the air, swinging both arms down while spreading them out to touch the ground as well. Jump back into the starting position by bringing both feet together. Repeat as many times as you like.

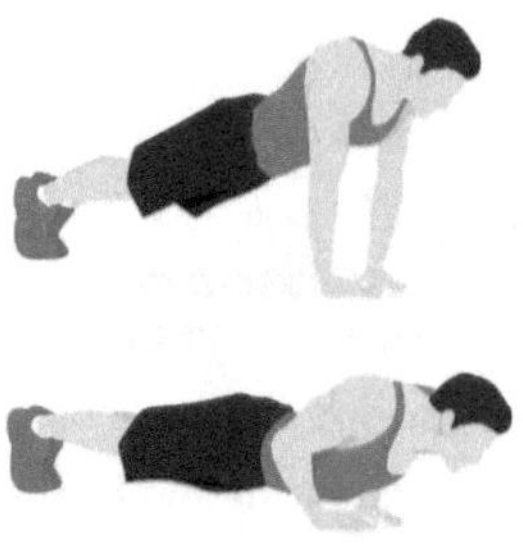

**#7: Triceps Push-Up:** The triceps push-up is a great exercise for improving upper body strength and toning your triceps. It can be done on any surface, but is usually done with a bench. To do this, lower yourself down until your arms are straight with hands facing forward, then push yourself back up. Repeat as many times as you like.

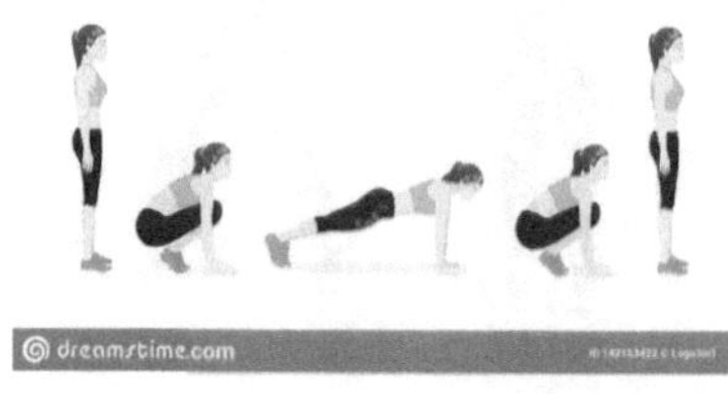

**#8: Squat Thrusts:** The squat thrust is an exercise that can be done at home or in the gym. To do this, lay face down on the ground with your arms by your side and feet together. Then, slowly lift your both legs off the floor and hold them for 1 second. As you do this, throw your hands back behind you. Next, bring both feet back down to the ground as you jump up into the air. Repeat as many times as you like.

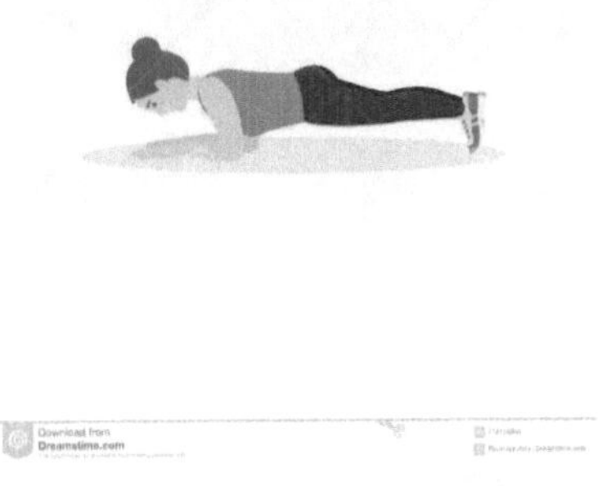



**#9: Plank:** The plank is another great exercise to improve strength and balance. For this exercise, you'll need a flat surface to lay on. Start through laying down on your stomach with arms and elbows by your sides. Then, straighten your legs out behind you so that you're in a plank position. Hold the position for 30 seconds, then switch sides for another 30 seconds. Repeat as many times as you like.

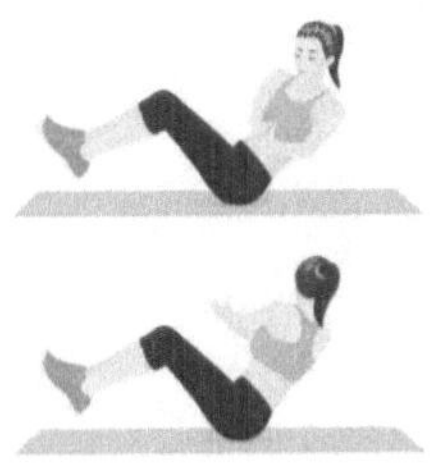

**#10: The Twist:** The twist is an exercise that can be done anywhere with a full water bottle. Simply grab the bottle by the neck with both hands and lift it to your chest while keeping your hips flat on the ground. Then, twist your body so that you face the opposite direction as your arms go over to the left and right. Repeat as many times as you like.

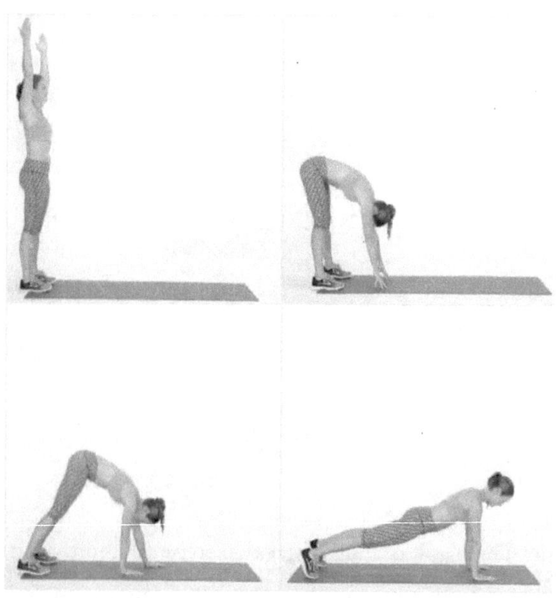

**#11: Walk-Out:** The walk-out is a great exercise that can be done by yourself or in a group at home. To do this, stand tall and bend at the knees so that your legs are bent at 90 degrees. Then, just kick one leg out to the side while keeping the other one straight behind you. Repeat as many times as you like.

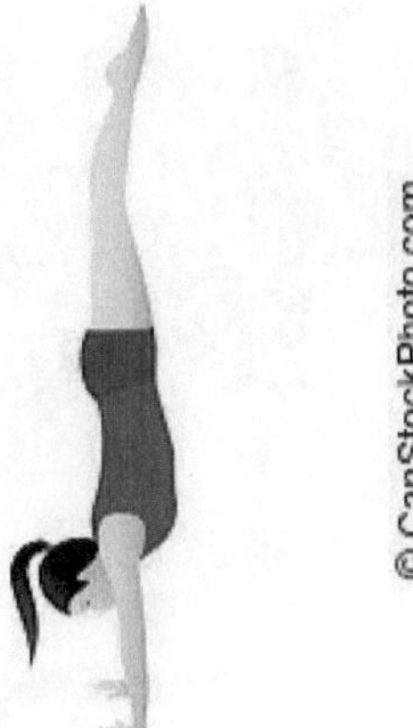

#12: **Handstand:** The handstand kick is an exercise that can be done by yourself or with a partner. If you're doing it by yourself, make sure to have a wall to lean against. To do this, just put your hands on the ground in front of you with your legs straightened behind you. Then, kick up into a handstand (chest facing the ground). Once you get there, jump up and down as many times as you can before dropping back down into a standing position. Repeat this as many reps as you like.

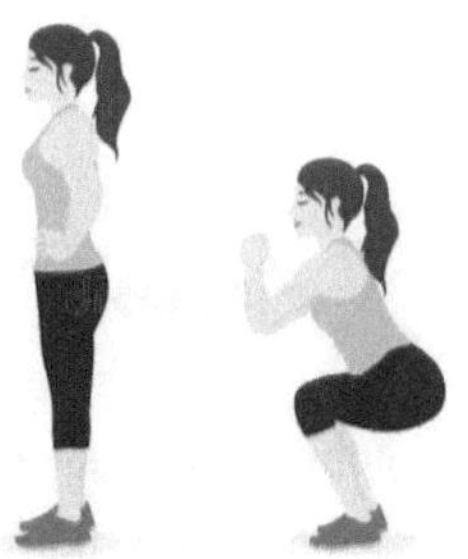

#13: **Squat with a Push:** The squat with push is an exercise that can be done anywhere. To do this, perform a regular squat with your hands on the back of your knees and then, kick out to the side while pushing out against the ground with both hands. Repeat as many times as you like.

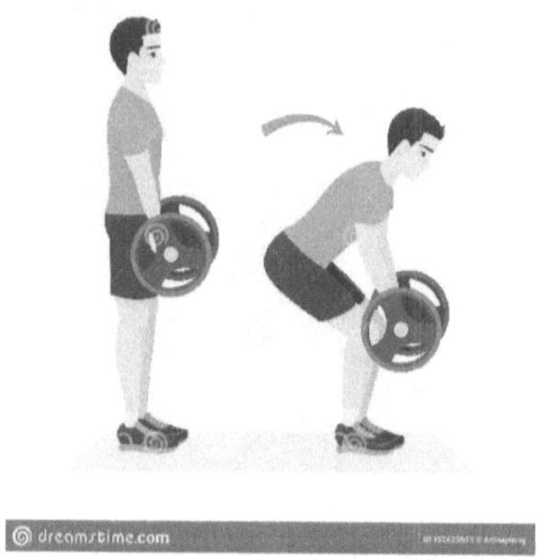

**#14: Deadlift:** The deadlift is an exercise that can be done anywhere. To do this, stand up straight with your feet together and hands on your hips. Then, bend at the knees so that your thighs are parallel to the ground. Next, hinge at the hips and lower yourself, bending at the waist but keeping your back and legs straight. Stand up as you push off through the floor with your legs. Repeat as many times as you like.

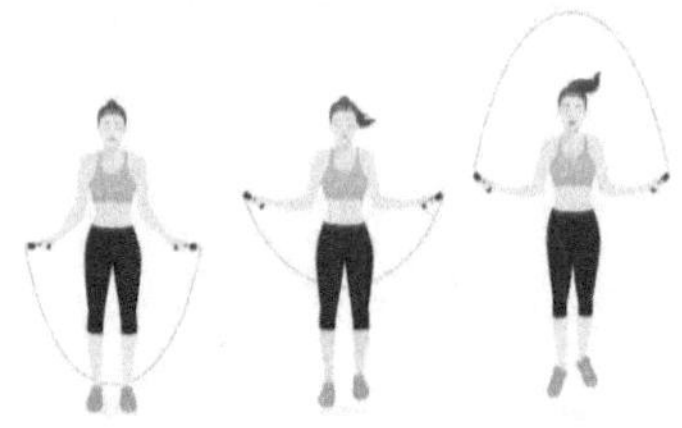

**#15: Jump Rope:** The jump rope is an exercise that can be done anywhere with a rope that's about 8 feet long. Start by standing next to the rope with your feet together. Then, start bouncing up and down on one foot while pulling the other one along next to you. Do this as many times as you can while maintaining a steady pace.

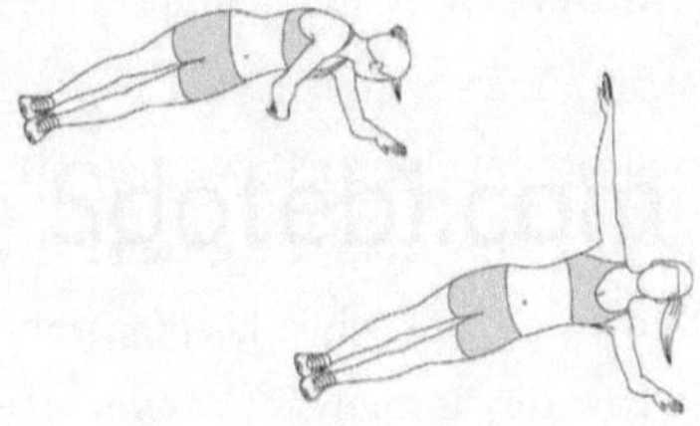

**#16: Plank with Twist:** The plank with a twist is an exercise that can be done anywhere. To do this, just get into a plank position as shown above. Then, turn to the side with your torso while keeping your hips still. Twist gently as you return to the starting position. Repeat on both sides for as many reps as you like.

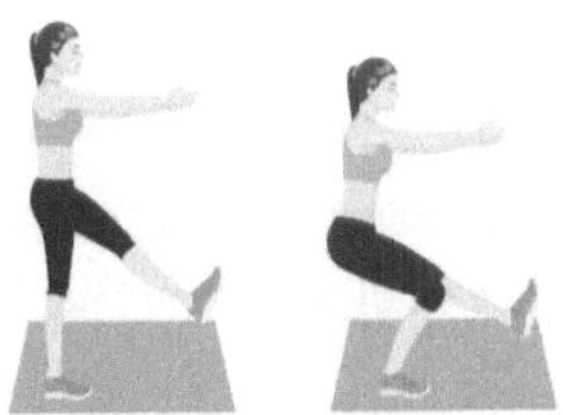

**#17: One-Legged Squat:** The one-legged squat is an exercise that can be done anywhere with a chair or stool. To do this, just stand on one leg and hold onto a chair behind you for balance. Then, bend over and lower yourself down into a squat with the other leg still in place. Return to standing up and repeat as many times as you like.

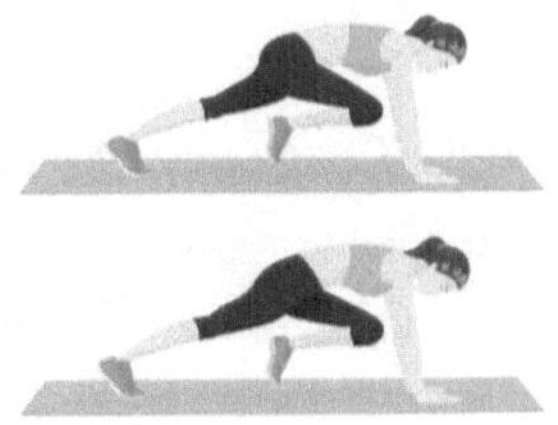

**#18: Mountain Climbers:** Mountain climbers are an exercise that can be done anywhere with a mat or thin mat. Lay down on your stomach and then raise yourself up onto one elbow, then place the other on the ground while raising your hips from the ground as well. Bring that leg that's on the ground to your chest while keeping your other foot planted flat on the ground. Repeat this as many reps as you like.

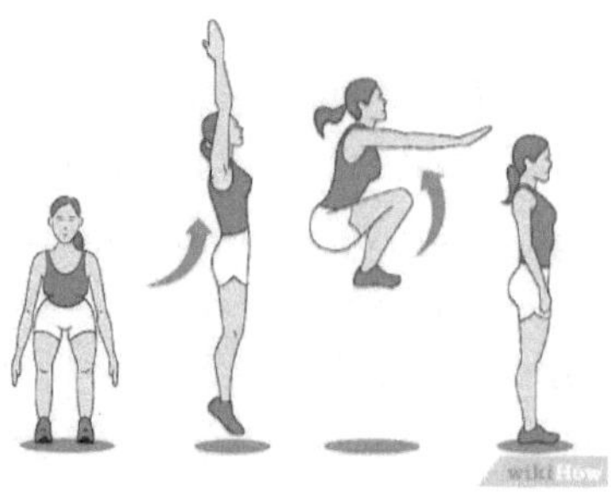

**#19: Plyometrics:** Plyometrics is an exercise that can be done anywhere with a mini-trampoline. Lay on the tray and jump up into the air as high as you can while landing on your feet. Do this as many times as you like.

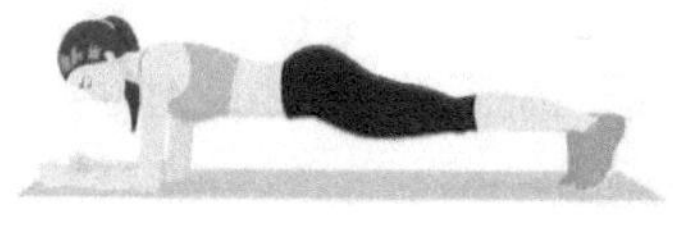

shutterstock.com · 323912273

**#20: Plank with a Punch:** The plank with a punch is an exercise that can be done anywhere with a bed or anything hard. To do this, just get into a plank position as shown above. Then, punch out on both sides one after another while keeping your core tight. Repeat as many times as you like.

Home exercises for beginners are absolutely necessary because they don't require any equipment or a gym membership. If you're trying to get your body into shape and you don't have a lot of money, doing these exercises at home is a great way to get there.

## HOW TO LOSE WEIGHT WITH HOME EXERCISES?

The great way to lose weight is to get rid of the things you eat that are unhealthy and replace them with healthy alternatives. The problem is we know that it can be difficult, if not impossible, to achieve weight loss without a dedicated time and effort. This section will walk you through some proven methods for getting in shape without dropping your activity level or going on an extreme diet.

The first strategy is a circuit training program where you do ten reps of each exercise continuously before moving on to another one. This is a very effective way to burn the maximum number of calories in the shortest amount of time. An example of a circuit would be to start with one foot in front of the other, hands on hips, and then do ten pushups. Once you complete that move to planking with your arms extended out in front of you for ten reps. from there move to crunches for ten reps and finally finish with ten squats. This is just an example but this style can be used with other exercises as well.

The next way is doing cardio before or after your weightlifting routine. This will be the same exercise for both as you might have figured but it helps you burn even more calories and puts your heart to work. So, if you are already doing weight training every day try adding in a twenty minute jog before or right after your workout. If this is too much you can also try walking for half an hour on days when you don't lift weights and increase the intensity as you get more fit.

The next strategy is to increase the volume and intensity of your workouts. The basic idea behind this is that you continue to do the same exercise throughout your routine until your body becomes used to the movement and then start adding in new variations and exercises. With circuit training that means doing ten reps of each exercise before moving on to another one. This way, you will be getting more work out but burning more calories at the same time. This method also works well for weightlifting as you will be adding in different muscle groups with every set.

The next tip is to eat less frequently, but more food at each meal. If you have smaller meals more times per day your body will be burning constantly and you will not store calories as fat. This also means that you must eat more healthy foods at each meal and not just junk and processed foods.

The last strategy is to do more cardiovascular exercise. If you have been doing weight training for a while you will start to lose muscle mass and strength. This is not a problem because you can replace lost muscle with leaner tissue but it will take longer for your body to get used to the action of lifting weights again and regain the speed and power which your muscles had before. For this reason, it makes sense to add in some cardio workouts into your schedule.

Although losing weight is important, exercise is even more critical in slowing aging. There are some different ways to boost your exercise regime. One is to buy the right equipment such as treadmills and stationary bicycles. These machines provide a safe environment for you work out in, but this does not mean that you should recklessly use them without any regard for your health. Another way to improve your exercise routine is by keeping a journal of how many times you exercise every day. This will help you keep track of what is working well and what needs improvement.

# HOW TO GET STRONGER WITH HOME EXERCISE?

The stronger we are, the better we'll feel. It may not appear worth the effort, but home exercises can make a world of difference in our daily lives and make us feel stronger and more confident. We'll be able to do more with less effort - work longer hours, take on heavier tasks, and enjoy our favorite hobbies without getting so tired. Most of us are not capable to do a full-time job and still be strong. We might work out when we can, but our time is limited so we have to make the most of the time we have. The best way to use your workout time is to add home exercises into it. You'll get in your exercise while watching TV, reading a book, or making dinner. You'll be able to work out at any time of day or night and it'll feel effortless.

*Why do home exercises?*

A lot of folks think they should go to the gym for strength training. That's great if you're able to do it, but the truth is that it takes a lot of time to get in the workout and then travel there. How many of us really have time for that? You could save time by doing home exercises during your lunch break. Most jobs will even let you take a short break so you can have your time and still be productive at work, too. In fact, you'll be happier and more productive if you exercise because you'll have more energy throughout the day.

Home exercises are meant to complement a regular workout routine. For example, if your usual workout is two days per week, add in another day with home exercises. You can do this on the off days or you can even do them twice a day on those days in order to make sure that your whole body gets worked out. Some people gravitate towards doing home exercises in the morning and then again at night. That's fine too, as long as you don't forget about them during the week.

There are many types of home exercises - some are focused on a partic- ular muscle or muscle group while others will work multiple muscles at the same time. Please note that not all of the exercises are appropriate for everyone, so consider your body type and your physical limitations when selecting an exercise. Also, try to select exercises that you enjoy so that you can get the most out of your workout routine!

*How to do home exercises*

It's very important that you don't get frustrated with your exercise routine. You should push yourself, but not too hard and not so often that you get injured. Everyone responds a little differently to the same exercises, and if you start doing them too often or too intensely, you can lose the benefits. You'll want to start at a level that's comfortable for you, and work your way up over time.

If you have any doubts or questions, consult with your doctor before doing a home exercise.

If it's easy to do an exercise, you probably need to make it harder. You'll be able to add more resistance (weights, resistance bands, or ankle weights) as you get stronger.

You should spend at least 15 minutes working out each time and no longer than 45 minutes. Don't forget about your warm up! A good warm up means you'll have less chance of injury and will get the most out of your workout.

Here are some good home exercises to try:

**Chest:** Push-ups (hands on the floor, feet on a bench or chair), bench press, chest press.
**Legs:** Squats, lunges, standing calf raise.
Shoulders: Overhead press (hands in front of shoulders), arnoid raise (arms out to the side).
**Back and Biceps:** Pull ups (chin up bar or pull up bar or chair), dead lift, bicep curl (with hand weights).

**Triceps and Arms:** Triceps extensions (bench or chair), overhead press (hands on an object), bicep curl.

There's a lot of other exercises that you can do to build your strength and stamina. Just follow the basic principles listed above and you'll be able to take control of your health and wellness.

# 3

# HOME WORKOUT ROUTINES FOR MEN AND WOMEN

Getting in shape and becoming healthier is easier than you think. If it's time to start working on your fitness, don't sweat it! There are plenty of ways to get into shape without ever leaving the comfort of your home. Getting healthy and fit is all about making little changes over time that add up to big improvements. Try our at-home workout tips to increase your endurance and build strength.

Here are some great home exercises that you can do to increase your daily calorie burn and stamina:

**Floor sit-ups:** These are classic exercises that will work out your abs. Lay straight on the floor, keeping your hands behind your head, and hold at the top of each sit-up. Do this exercise for a total of 50 repetitions in three sets with 10 seconds rest between each set.

**Plank position:** This is another great exercise for strengthening your midsection. Lay on the floor, keeping your body in a straight line. Hold for 30 seconds.

**Pushups:** Pushups are easy and great if you don't have any equipment. You can execute this on your knees or with your feet on a raised surface.

You can do this as many as you can, then rest and repeat the exercise three times.

**Leg raises:** Another great exercise for the abs, you can do this by laying on your back, keeping your arms straight up overhead and flexing your legs straight up. Do 20-25 leg raises with 10 seconds of rest between each exercise.

**Squats:** These are a great move if you lack equipment. Your legs shoulder width apart then hold your body weight and squat down until you go below parallel, then get back to standing position. Do 10 repetitions with a 30-second break in between each set.

**Lunges:** Stand up straight with your legs and arms shoulder-width apart and lunge forward. Once you go down with one knee, bend down as far as you can with your front knee. Alternate legs after the first set.

**Plank:** Lay on the floor with two hands directly below your shoulder and raise yourself up on all fours. Hold for 30 seconds then rest, then repeat three times.

**Stretches:** Stretching is an important part of any workout. You should stretch before and after working out with weights or other forms of exercise. Stretch for 10-15 seconds at a time, holding each stretch for a few seconds.

**Pushups:** This is another great move if you have no equipment. Do pushups by laying on your stomach, lifting your body up with your arms straight out in front of you and lifting yourself back down until your arms are straight again. You can do this as many as you can, then rest and repeat the exercise three times.

**Seated Leg Raises:** These are great for your abs and hips. Sit on the floor with your legs straight out in front of you, bend your back leg at the knee and keep it flexed, lift up straight out of the chair. Lift your arms until parallel with the floor. Do this for 20-25 reps with a 30-second rest between each set.

These are a few different exercises that you can do at home. Try to work on a different one each day and increase the reps for a week, then move on to something new. It's easy to get into shape at home. Don't forget to stretch and drink lots of water!

## THE BEST KIND OF DIET PLAN FOR HOME WORKOUT ROUTINES

Diets are always hard. They're restrictive, and sometimes you just don't know how to follow them. And then there are the workouts! They require us to get out of our houses and do something we don't want to be doing anyway, even if it means going out in public with our sweaty selves. But all that being said, there's one kind of home workout routine and diet plan for home workout routines.

The Best Kind of Diet Plan for Home Workout Routines:

- At the beginning of every week, weigh yourself. This is called your weight baseline. On your scale, the number is useless, so write it down on a piece of paper. On that same piece of paper, insert how much weight you want to lose or how much weight you want to gain. That'll motivate you to get started on your diet.
- Find your routine. Figure out a regular time of day to exercise. Make sure you get your exercise in the morning so that your metabolism is working at its highest during the rest of the day.
- Set a goal. Each week, set a new goal to lose or gain weight. For example, if you want to lose weight, set your goal at a pound a week. Once you've reached that goal, go up by another twenty-five pounds for the next one. Set a goal to have abs. It will not be easy, but it can lead to a lot of self-confidence.
- Create a meal plan. Meal planning is the initial principle of healthy eating. If you prepare such nutritious meals and snacks in advance you'll be less likely to lure of processed meals and fast

food. You could even use the time you save by prepping your meals to fit in more exercise. To begin this, try to search for recipes that align with your diet of choice. Find a few meals that you find appetizing and create a list of groceries. When you're at the store, stick to your list only. Following a successful grocery shopping trip, and set aside an hour or two to prep your meals all at once. Chopping produce and then cooking grains in advance will help you save valuable time during the week.

- Go shopping for groceries. You'll need a notebook or journal to keep track of the calories and nutrients you consume and how much exercise you get. Try to get a nutritionist's advice on what you should be eating and how much exercise you should get.

- Use the calories you consume as a means of motivation. Cut down on the junk food and alcohol you consume. Avoid eating out at restaurants whose calorie counts you can't figure out and don't expect a lot of processed foods or candy to be available.

- Eat a mix of proteins and carbs every day. Protein is used for muscle recovery and energy production while carbohydrates are used to replenish energy supplies that have been depleted.

- Carbohydrates are an important part of your diet, but you should still monitor how many of them you eat. Carbohydrates are essential for muscle growth. If you take in too few carbs, you won't be able to build new muscle tissue.

- Protein is also important for building muscle, but you should avoid overdoing it. If you eat too much protein, your muscles won't be able to absorb enough protein to build new muscle.

- For workouts, eat your pre-workout meal two to four hours before. For example, if your workout begins at 8:30 a.m., then you should eat your pre-workout meal around 6:30 a.m. or even earlier in order to allow for digestion time before the workout.

- During the actual workout, drinking 2 to 4 ounces of water will help you stay hydrated as well as give you a little energy boost. Whatever you do, avoid soda and sugary drinks like regular coffee.

- Eat smaller portions every three hours. This will allow your body to have enough energy to work out.
- Make sure you drink plenty of water after each workout. Exercising in the heat is even more important than exercising in cold weather because it can dehydrate your body faster.

The best diet plan can help us get fit and healthy. It is important that we get the correct diet, exercise, and drink enough water. If we don't have these, then our bodies won't have the energy to exercise and will be more prone to diseases and health problems. It can also help us achieve a nice body at any age. This way, we will feel comfortable about ourselves and be able to live longer with less pain from diseases such as arthritis or diabetes.

Go through this process every day and see how much you can do. It will definitely add up to more than anything if you're consistent. Having a routine also helps us stick to the diet plan we have developed. Having a routine keeps us on track, so if you want to develop a healthy lifestyle, find out what works best for you, follow the best diet plan and stay consistent with it.

## BENEFITS OF HEALTHY EATING

An improvement in health and the quality of life is what motivates many people to start a new diet or start working out. As well, there are other benefits that could be discovered through doing an adequate amount of exercise at home. A healthy diet, and a balanced exercise regimen will help to improve the quality of life of the people who have made this change. A healthy diet is consists of, fruits, vegetables, lean proteins, and whole grains. These foods are very rich in vitamins, minerals, and other nutrients that are needed for the body to function properly. After some time of eating healthy, you will start to notice that your energy levels are increasing and your mind is functioning better. If you choose to add exercise into your daily plan, this can be a great way to burn off calories and fat while giving yourself a boost of energy. Here are some of the benefits that can be discovered from participating in a healthy diet and exercise program.

### Burning off the excess calories

Burning off the excess calories that you consume will prevent additional fat from being absorbed into your body. If you are able to burn off the extra calories, you will be able to maintain your desired weight or continue to lose weight.

### Prevent the risk of developing heart disease

Another benefit of a healthy diet is that it can help prevent the risk of developing heart disease. A healthy diet can promote a lean body mass while also lowering your blood cholesterol levels. Exercise can also decrease the risk of heart disease, and it will also help to lower blood pressure.

### Handling chronic diseases

It is also possible to handle some of the chronic diseases that have been developing over time with a healthy diet and exercise program. Diabetes, blood pressure issues, and obesity are some of the chronic diseases that can be improved with both a healthy diet and an exercise program.

If you decide to make these positive changes in your life, you can get rid of the extra fat, see better health, and feel great about yourself. You won't regret the changes that you make, and your body will thank you for the boost of energy that you are introducing into it.

## VARIETIES OF FOOD SHOULD YOU EAT FOR A HEALTHY DIET

You should change your diet to a healthy diet to get fit at home. The healthy diet should be made up of organic and fresh foods. These foods should be high in fiber, low in fat, and have the right amount of protein.

First, start your day with a whole grain like oatmeal or toast with peanut butter on it. The digestion of whole grains takes a longer time for the body to break down, so you stay fuller longer. Avoid white bread and white rice because they are simple carbohydrates and cause spikes in insulin levels. Eating organic food is recommended because they have higher amounts of fiber than processed foods, plus they are low in fat and sugar.

Second, eat a lot of fruits and vegetables. Fruits and vegetables contain antioxidants which are good for your immune system. Eat one serving per meal such as a salad or any other vegetable dishes with low-fat dressing.

Third, drink eight glasses of water a day. Hydration is crucial to your body because it helps your metabolism and digestion, which in turn helps speed up the body's fat burning process. Water contains no calories and it is also a great way to lose weight.

Fourth, eat lean meats like turkey breast and chicken breast. Lean protein helps build muscle mass in the body whereas fatty meats increase fat storage in your body. The recommended amount of protein each day for women is 46 grams and 64 grams for men.

Fifth, eat whole grains like quinoa, barley, millet and buckwheat. Whole grains are rich with fiber and make you feel full longer. They are also high in antioxidants and alpha-linolenic acid which is an omega-3 fat. Avoid refined grains like white rice because they are simple carbohydrates that cause spikes in insulin levels.

Sixth, eat plenty of nuts and seeds. Nuts and seeds have high amounts of protein while being low in fat. They provide a good amount of monounsaturated fats which help lower cholesterol.

## HOME WORKOUT ROUTINES FOR YOGA AND PILATES

Yoga is a form of exercise that helps with flexibility, breathing, and more. Yoga exercises are meant to be done on the floor because this provides the leverage you need to balance yourself. It is a great workout for focusing your mind on deep breathing while stretching muscles in the body, as well as temperature regulation through poses involving bends and twists (asanas).

According to studies, learning yoga has made people to be more calm, sleep better and feel healthier. And the most important thing is how you believe in it. Because it is said that if you believe in the power of yoga, you will get the best results.

On the other hand, Pilates is an exercise system that focuses on improving strength, flexibility and coordination of muscles through a series of specific, continuous movements. The fundamental principle behind Pilates is to develop core strength by focusing on the muscles of the stomach, back and trunk. While some mat work does include stretching of the limbs, its main focus is strengthening the deeper abdominal muscles along with pelvic floor control.

**Home workout routines for yoga:**

What you need: 1 mat, 1 cushion and a wall

*Instructions 1:* Lie face up on the floor using the cushion under your head, bend your knees and place your feet flat on the floor. Relax, breathe deeply in and out. Fold your right knee into your chest using both hands to hold it there while you exhale. Repeat this for 10 times.

*Instructions 2:* Do not move too fast with this exercise as you have to stretch it as much as possible. Get yourself in a sitting position with your legs extended, clasping your hands around the feet and pulling backwards for a gentle stretch. Repeat this for ten times.

*Instructions 3:* Lie face up on the floor using the cushion under your head, stretch both legs straight out while you place both hands at the back of your head. Do this exercise while breathing deeply in and out. You can try this exercise with one leg at a time to stretch it better and repeat it for 10 times each leg.

*Instructions 4:* Lie face up on the floor using the cushion under your head, extend both legs out and put your hands behind your head. Do this for 10 to 12 times.

*Instructions 5:* Lie face up on the floor using the cushion under your head, keeping both hands at sides as well as legs straight out, breathe deeply in and out while you can try this exercise with one leg at a time to stretch it better and repeat it for 10 times each leg.

*Instructions 6:* Lie face up on the floor using the cushion under your head, with legs out and knees straight. Extend both arms out in front for balance. Do this exercise while breathing deeply in and out. You can try this exercise with one leg at a time to stretch it better and repeat it for 10 times each leg.

*Instructions 7:* Lie face up on the floor using the cushion under your head, extend both legs out while you put both hands behind your head. Do this exercise while breathing deeply in and out.

*Instructions 8:* Lie face up on the floor using the cushion under your head, bend both legs and put your hands at your back. Do this exercise while breathing deeply in and out.

*Instructions 9:* Lie face up on the floor using the cushion under your head, bend both knees and place both hands at the back of your neck.

*Instructions 10:* Lie face up on the floor with a cushion under your head, extend both legs straight out and place both arms underneath you as if you are lifting yourself off the ground.

These yoga exercises should be done for three weeks in a row or more. You can do three sets of 10 to 12 repetitions each exercise.

## Home workout routines for Pilates:

This set of Pilate's exercises is designed to provide you with a total body workout that includes stability, endurance and flexibility. It is great to do these exercises in the morning as it gets your metabolism going for the day. 15 minutes of Pilates is fun and effective and best of all, you can do it at home without extra equipment.

**What you need:** 1 mat

*Instructions 1:* Place your mat on the floor in front of a wall. Lie face down on the mat then your arms by your sides and your legs extended out behind you. Raise both legs off the floor and bend at your knees to lower them toward the floor. As you exhale, squeeze one knee into the chest to bring it back to start position and repeat with opposite leg. Do this exercise for 10 times with each leg.

*Instructions 2:* Lie face down on the mat with your arms by your sides and your legs extended out behind you. Stretch both legs out in front. Keep the left leg straight and bend the right knee to lower it toward the floor as you equalize it with the right leg. Then, pull the right knee back into starting position as you inhale and repeat for 10 times.

*Instructions 3:* Lie face down on the mat with your arms by your sides and your legs extended out behind you. Keeping both legs straight, bend at the knees to lower them toward the floor to start position. Inhale and exhale as you pull back up and keep your legs straight. Repeat for 10 times.

*Instructions 4:* Lie face down on the mat with your arms by your sides and your legs extended out behind you. Raise both legs off the floor and bend at the knees to lower them toward the floor. As you exhale, squeeze one knee into the chest to bring it back to start position and repeat with opposite leg. Do this exercise for 10 times with each leg.

*Instructions 5:* Lie face down on the mat with your arms by your sides and your legs extended out behind you. Keeping both legs straight, extend out both arms in front of you. Then, bend both knees to lower them toward the floor. Inhale and exhale as you pull back up and keep your legs straight. Repeat for 10 times.

*Instructions 6:* Lie face down on the mat with your arms by your sides and your legs extended out behind you. Keeping both legs straight, lift both arms back behind you. Bend your both knees at the same time to lower them toward the floor to start position. Inhale and exhale as you pull back up and keep your legs straight. Repeat for 10 times.

These Yoga exercises should be done for three weeks in a row or more. You can do three sets at ten time for each exercise.

If you want to get fit, lose weight and improve your health, both yoga and Pilate's exercises should be a part of your physical fitness routine. Both of these exercises will help you in your goal to get fit. Pilates is a great exercise to build core strength while yoga will stretch and tone all the muscles in your body.

In summary, both yoga and Pilates could help you to get fit and stay fit for a lifetime. As we have seen, yoga helps you build physical strength, flexibility and mental agility for better performance. Pilates is a great way to firm and tone the muscles in your body so that you can be healthy and strong from within. When performed regularly, these exercises could help you live a life free of illnesses and disease.

In short, yoga and Pilates do not only make you look good but make you feel good too. Don't miss out on these dynamic workouts, get fit now and start living healthily!

# 4

# FUN HOME EXERCISES

Many people find it difficult to start an exercise routine but these exercises can be easily done at home. With fun home exercises, you can enjoy a well-balanced, and healthy lifestyle. It is also an important part of a healthy life.

Fun Home Exercises are a great way for you to get the exercise you want and need without taking up too much time. They provide an opportunity for people to exercise in the privacy of their homes without having to worry about being outside, sweating, or getting a sunburn.

The biggest benefit to Fun Home Exercises is that they provide a way for people to exercise in the convenience of their own homes, when it is convenient for them. Because going to the gym can be inconvenient for some people and having a difficult schedule can also make it hard for some people to get out of the house and do things, therefore having at home fun exercises provide an easy alternative.

While fun exercises are beneficial for people, they are also essential for many other reasons. These exercises provide an opportunity for people to relieve the stress and anxiety from everyday life. These can also ease chronic pain and help people get in touch with their bodies again after a long illness.

Fun Home Exercises also improve the self-esteem and confidence of the people who use them. This means more people are likely to exercise on their homes, than get a gym membership, because they feel more confident.

## THE IMPORTANCE OF HAVING FUN WHILE YOU EXERCISE

Having fun while you exercise is important for a number of reasons. First of all, studies have shown that laughter improves your blood circulation. It also improves your mood and also reduces stress. And it strengthens the immune system. Having fun while you exercise is important not only to improve your health but also to make time fly by faster so that you don't dread working out!

Secondly, it releases endorphins, which give you an overall sense of well-being. Endorphins are the "feel good" hormones that we all desire for ourselves after exercising. These endorphins also have an effect on our muscles. When you exercise, your muscles are under a lot of stress, so they need to be given food and oxygen in order to repair themselves and grow new fibers. Endorphin production can help this process along, making you stronger, better looking, and feeling better than ever after you're finished working out. It also helps you to keep your mind focused on what you're doing instead of thinking about other things.

Thirdly, it keeps you interested in doing your exercise routine. By having fun while you exercise, you will stimulate your brain very well. If you're doing something that interests you, then it's very likely that your brain will learn more. This is especially true if the activity requires some sort of mental strain and focus like intense weightlifting or other high-intensity exercises.

Fourthly, there are many experts who say that exercise and laughter go hand in hand because they improve your mood to such an extent that it results in a higher level of performance during both activities.

Laughter improves the mental aspects of your fitness. Having fun while you exercise will improve your concentration and your focus if you are in a sports-related activity, because you will be stimulating the "frontal lobes" of your brain; the part associated with logic, problem solving, and decision making.

Lastly, it helps you reach your training goals. There are a lot of different reasons to exercise, but the main one is to become healthier and looking better physically. This can be accomplished with regular workouts. However, if you don't find it enjoyable, you will be unable to stick with it and may eventually give up on your fitness goals altogether.

People who exercise with a smile on their face are more likely to achieve fitness goals and stay active than those who are not and you can boost your energy levels and mood by over 50%. The neurotransmitter serotonin helps the body release feelings of pleasure and enhances the social experience of exercising. If you are someone who finds running or any other type of workout pretty dull, then try to spice it up with some laughter. And of course, it is a must to make the most of exercise while you are on the move.

You may believe that you are providing your body with a workout session, but in reality, it's also offering you a mental workout. Remember that having fun while exercising benefits both your physical and mental health. No matter what your fitness level is, you can always add some fun to your next exercise routine. There are many ways to make exercising more enjoyable. For example, instead of running on a treadmill in front of the TV, try watching a comedy show or listening to your favorite music while running on the treadmill. This will not only allow you to have more fun while exercising but will also make it easier to keep your motivation high and stay motivated for long-term results.

No matter what kind of exercise you want to get into, there are a number of ways to make it more enjoyable and fun so that you can keep improving over time.

## HOME EXERCISES FOR CHILDREN

There are various great exercises that can be done at home which will help to increase your fitness and flexibility. They can be done by your children or just as a way to help keep their body healthy that you can teach your child and do together!

1. Stand up and then stretch forward from the waist, palms on the floor maintaining balance with arms extended. Slowly bend knees lowering body towards the ground while breathing out, hold the position for 1-2 seconds, and then slowly come back to starting position while breathing in. Hold for a second and repeat the exercise again. Do it around 5-10 times.

2. Squat down as if to sit on a chair, hold the position for a second and then come back to the standing position of course without sitting on a chair. Then repeat this for 5-10 times.

3. Stand up straight with palms together in front of the chest, then slowly move hands forward and backward while breathing in and out respectively. Do it around 10-15 times and then relax.

4. Bring both hands to your chest and squeeze it tightly, you will feel pressure. Do this for a few times and then relax.

5. Lift both hands behind your head; do this for holding the head in place. Then bend forward while breathing out and then lift shoulder up, hold the position for a second and repeat 5-10 times.

6. Running. Although it may appear simple, chasing each other around is one of the most beneficial activities for children. Running is particularly healthy for your kids since it helps them build strong bones while strengthening their muscles. Not to mention, it's fun to run. Coupled with a healthy diet, it also helps

children maintain a healthy weight. Children can develop a love of running and seeing it as a joyful activity it is something that they can carry into adulthood, setting them up for a lifetime of healthy habits.

7. Supermans. Lie on your stomach, arms extended, legs out behind you, and raise both arms and legs together off the ground while breathing in. Hold the position for a second and repeat 10-15 times. They are also a great got improving the vestibular system of children.

8. Leg Raises. Lie down on your back, straighten your knees so your feet are off the floor. Lift both feet off the floor simultaneously holding for a second and then come back to starting position while breathing out. Do it around 10-15 times and then relax.

9. The Dancing Plank. This is a fun one to do together and doesn't require much space at all! Begin in a plank position with your hands underneath of you on the ground, then tap one hand out to the side and return it back under you while tapping out the other hand. Do it around 5-10 times and then switch sides.

Exercises are good for children to do to help build and maintain healthy minds and bodies. It also helps children get active which is important for their overall development. Getting your child involved in some type of activity is a great way to help them grow into a healthy adult and will build their confidence. Safety is the most important thing!

## HOW TO MAKE YOUR HOME EXERCISES FUN AND ENGAGING?

Many people find it hard to get motivated when it comes to exercise. When the window of opportunity closes, they usually resort back to working out in the gym or routine sets of monotonous exercises.

However, there are plenty of ways for you and your body to stay active without a full-fledged workout. You can make your exercises fun by working on things that are relevant to your daily life, like an arm curl while talking on the phone or a long jump while folding laundry. Not only will these activities get you in the habit of working out, they will also be more pleasant and with these ideas, you can do away with a pointless workout routine.

*How to make your home exercises fun and engaging? Follow these steps:*

1. Do a few deep stretches before every workout session.
2. Listen to music while doing the exercises. It will help you get in the zone, and it will make your routine more like a dance party than an exercise session.
3. Make it a game! Make it a goal to improve your form and increase the intensity of each move over time. You'll be surprised by how addictive this can be!
4. Keep a journal and track your progress. You'll be more inclined to stick with it if you know you're getting results.
5. Watch something like funny movie or TV show while doing the exercises.
6. Do a few exercises while talking on the phone, folding laundry, or surfing the internet...you choose!
7. Find some fun workout videos and watch them while working out in your home!
8. Create a home exercise routine that is specific to your needs. Your body is unique, so you should tailor your exercise sessions to meet your fitness needs.
9. Make home exercises fun with the help of some dance moves that you can do it in the living room, or try a few fun dance moves with an exercise ball.
10. Create your own workout playlist with some music you really like on it and listen to it as you get moving at home!

11. Dress up in workout clothes and dance around your living room to get your heart pumping! Just because you're dancing around the house doesn't mean it's not a good workout!

12. And of course...keep moving!

Home exercisers will never get bored doing the same things over and over again! At home exercising is always a different experience. These tips will make your exercises fun and engaging, and you'll be more likely to do them on a daily basis. A few quick exercises while doing chores around the house or a dance in the living room can do wonders for your workout routine.

# 5

# HOME EXERCISES FOR OLDER ADULTS

There are many benefits on maintaining a healthy lifestyle, but we all know that it's easier said than done. There's never enough time to go to the gym, exercise is boring, and no one wants to spend their day cooped up at home.

Getting older doesn't mean you can't stay active. In fact, exercise is even more important when you're older because it can help to reduce the risk of chronic diseases such as diabetes. In addition to improving your health, staying active improves your mood and can actually lead to a happier life.

At any age, it is important to be physically active. Physical inactivity is actually a serious public health problem for older adults because it can lead to heart disease, diabetes, high blood pressure and arthritis. These conditions may cause pain and stiffness that make it hard or impossible to stay active.

The good news is that it's never too late to start working out. With some tips and guidance from your doctor, you can get fit and healthy without making it seem like an unbearable chore.

Home exercise allows you to stay active while remaining sedentary. Most of us spend hours behind our computer or in front of our TV, so why not use that time to get in shape at home? Exercise done in time with your schedule, at home, becomes a means of staying healthy and maintaining a positive lifestyle.

Regular exercise helps build muscle tone and reduces weight gain when combined with proper eating habits. Regular exercise, combined with healthy eating habits, can help balance your weight and help curb the risk of many diseases including osteoporosis, heart problems, diabetes and high blood pressure.

The important thing about exercising that you must remember is to do the best you can. If you're not in good shape, don't try to do everything at once. Start with a little exercise every day - even just five minutes of walking can make a difference. Don't push yourself too hard, either. If you feel tired or out of breath, stop and rest.

If you do have pain that interferes with your activity level, talk to your doctor about the possible cause and treat the problem if you can. If not able to keep up your regular exercise routine, ask your doctor about any alternatives that could make it easier for you to get in shape, such as weight training or aerobic exercise.

There are a variety of exercises that you can perform at home alone or with the help of a friend, family member or partner. But, before you jump right in, it is very important to determine what type of exercise you prefer and how fit you have to be. If your goal is simply to stay in shape and maintain an ideal weight, then choose the easiest type of exercise for you.

## HOW TO MAINTAIN YOUR HOME EXERCISE ROUTINE THROUGHOUT LIFE?

Maintaining your home exercise routine throughout life can be difficult. However, there are a number of benefits to doing so.

It can help you stay in shape for your life. It can also aid in weight-loss and improve your posture. Furthermore, it might allow you to reduce your health care costs once you get older as if you don't have to be in the hospital as often.

Being fit at home is a good idea if you're looking for more ways to improve your life before reaching retirement age or just want something new that's different from exercising outside of the house. In addition, certain exercises like yoga and Pilates can relieve stress and help with sleeping better at night, both of which will add up over time and have long-lasting results for a healthier life.

In order to maintain your home exercise routine throughout life, there are several things that you should focus on doing on a regular basis. First, you should make sure that you're pushing yourself every day. Even if you can't complete all of the exercises you want to do, you should still try them occasionally. This way, it will be easier to pick them back up later on when things really start to get difficult and you're not able to do as much as you used to.

Next, it's important that you don't go overboard with any one exercise type. You should change things up from time to time and not stick to them too much. If you're finding it difficult to do any exercise, change it up by trying something else or start from a lower level that you're already comfortable with. You don't want to be too sore or tired either, especially if being fit at home is a new habit for you.

To avoid being too tired while working out, you should aim for between 45 and 60 minutes of exercise each day. Studies have shown that 30 minutes of exercise a day will typically give you the same results as 60 minutes, especially if you're more fit. When doing this at home, you can begin with 15 minutes and then add on to it if it's easy for you to do so.

Lastly, you should look into other ways to take care of yourself now that you're in your golden years. For example, it may be a good idea to start taking some supplements now so that they'll work better when your body starts falling apart later on. In addition, it might be time for you to change up your diet so that it's easier for you to eat healthy without feeling deprived all of the time. Maintaining your home exercise routine throughout life doesn't have to be difficult. However, you need to be careful not to overdo it on any one exercise type. If you're feeling good and having fun, it's probably going to last longer than if you're completely worn out all of the time.

You just have to make sure that you're doing both the exercises that are fun and entertaining for you as well as the ones that are guaranteed to keep you in shape throughout the years. That way, you can spend a little bit of time every day working out and still enjoy your life afterwards. It's all about finding what works best for you without sacrificing anything along the way.

In order to maintain your home exercise routine throughout life, it's a good idea for you to start thinking about what you can do when things get difficult or impossible in the future. This way, when your body starts slowing down in the future, you won't lose something that was really important to you.

## HOME EXERCISES FOR OLDER ADULTS: DIET, FITNESS, AND MEMORY IMPROVEMENT

The physical health and fitness benefits of exercise are unrivaled. Now, even in our older age, there is the option of home exercising which can be tailored to the individual needs.

This is a guide for how to create a simple routine that will have an immediate impact on your well-being. For those with arthritis or injuries, some exercises may not be possible. For everyone else, many of these exercises can easily be substituted with other movements that would still provide similar benefits without the risk of injury or strain on joints and muscles.

Visualize your exercise space. Whatever you are working out in, write down what it looks like. This will help you feel less awkward and more prepared when Step 2 comes around.

Begin with a warm-up routine of gentle stretching and range of motion exercises for the upper and lower body, including arms, wrists, shoulders and knees. Always consult your doctor to ensure exercises are appropriate for you; however, yoga is excellent for flexibility because it is done slowly and carefully so that people of all ages can participate. Additionally, yoga often incorporates meditation, which can reduce stress and improve memory.

Stretching is also beneficial as it prevents many muscle injuries and cramps that commonly occur during exercise in a home environment. If you do get injured abruptly, consult a doctor immediately.

If you are worried about the amount of time spent exercising, try to focus on how much better you feel afterward instead of how much time has passed.

The following exercises are complete body moves that are good for any age. Remember that these aren't meant to be quick, but slow and balanced. As you get older, it is especially important to move your body very slowly so that you don't injure yourself.

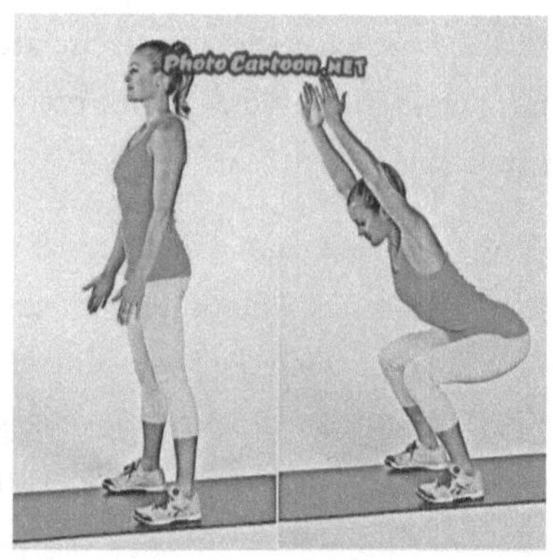

Squat and Reach: Stand with feet hip-width apart. Squat down as though you were about to sit in a chair until your thighs are parallel with the floor, keeping weight in the heels of your feet. As you stand back up, spread arms wide and reach as high as possible.

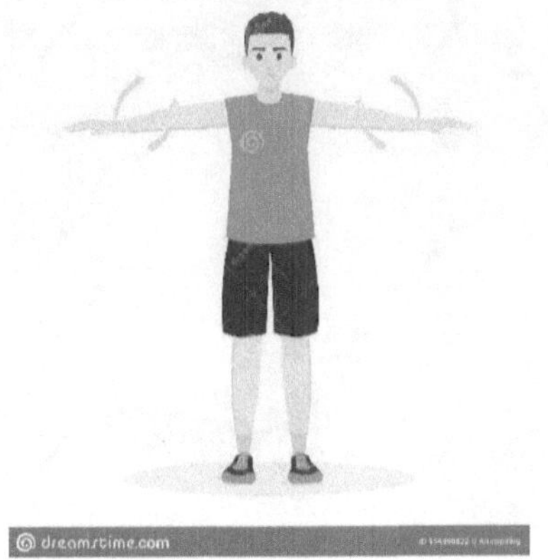

Standing arm rotation: Stand with feet about shoulder-width apart. Rotate arms in circles, one at a time, starting with the left arm and going clockwise three times. Then rotate the right arm counter-clockwise three times in a counter-clockwise direction. Think of this like stirring a bowl of soup upwards in a circular motion, drawing the soup to the tip of the spoon.

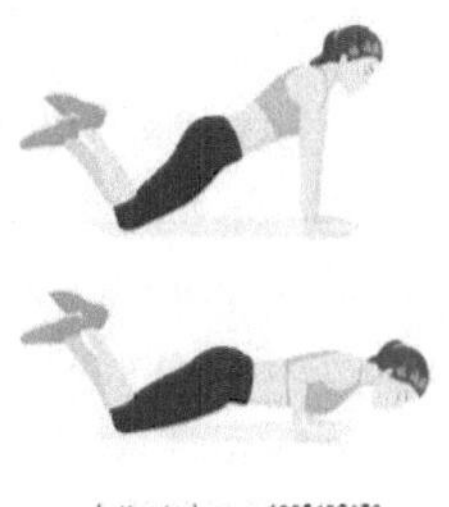

Push up and knee raise: Start with hands on the floor, palms facing down. Keep feet together and knees bent at a 90 degree angle. Push up so that arms are extended above the head while simultaneously lifting knees up to meet elbows. This counts as one repetition.

Repeat the circuit three times, depending on your fitness level and return to easy stretching for the rest of your body before moving on to your next exercise.

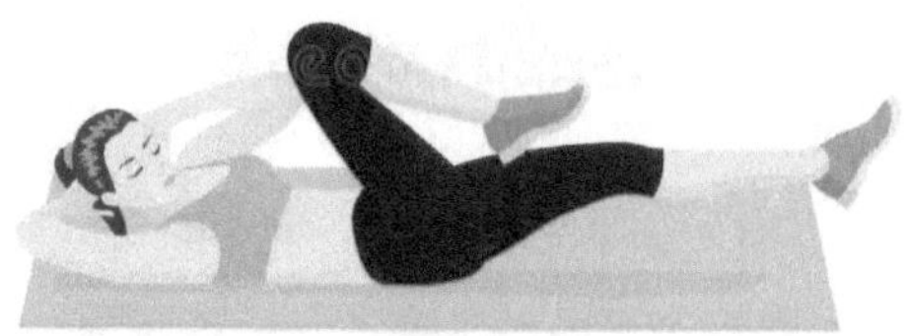

Bicycle Crunch: Place your hands behind your head and lay on a stability ball. Roll back to up with your right hand, rotating left leg out to the side. Place right hand on ground for support and stabilize left hand against hip.

You can burn calories in a little over an hour while using minimal space. It's not just for your muscles; it's also great for your lungs and heart. It is also low impact which means a reduced pressure on the joints.

Walking is also a great forms of exercise as it does not only strengthen the bones but also helps with weight loss and cardiovascular health. It is important to monitor your blood pressure to ensure that you do not become dehydrated or get lightheaded. If you are unsure if you can handle more intense exercise, consult a doctor first.

These are just several exercises to get you started, but really, the possibilities are endless. The point is to find what works for you and your body.

# 6

# HOW TO ENSURE THE SAFETY OF YOUR HOME EXERCISES

Whether you are looking to work out at home or maintain a healthy level of exercise, there's no reason for you not to use the right equipment. For many people, using equipment like exercise balls and step machines can be an awesome form of fun that can help with weight loss and physical fitness. To get the best result on your workout, you need to make sure that you don't injure yourself.

Doing the wrong kind of exercise at home can lead to injury. If you continue doing these exercises on a regular basis without making sure that they are correct and safe, it could lead to an injury. You should be careful when exercising in your home and make sure that it is well-maintained to avoid any type of accidents.

Exercising at home is great because you can be your own coach and create your own schedule. This is a nice change from needing to find time in your day to go to the gym. However, this doesn't mean that you will forget about using proper exercise form and supervising yourself at all times during the workout. It's important that you keep an eye out for any potential problems and resolve them before they become big issues. Make sure that you are moving properly to avoid hurting your joints.

## HOW TO KEEP HOME EXERCISING SAFE FOR EVERYONE.

To get the best out of your home exercise regime, it is important that you take into consideration safety. Incorporating safety into a routine can be as simple as taking precautions against injury and making sure that equipment is in good working order.

To help you get started on your home-exercise regime, here are some tips on safety in the home.

There are a number of areas to think about when it comes to safety at home. Firstly there are things such as equipment: is it in good condition or worn out? Is the equipment rated in kilograms or pounds? If so, make sure you know which weight rating system is used and that all the weights for the set are present and in good working order.

Beware of old equipment. Equipment that is old, especially if it has been passed down to you from your parents, grandparents and so on, may be unsafe to use. The material it is made from may rust or breakdown easily, causing injury and accidents.

Also be wary of using equipment that has become damaged or worn out due to neglect. For example, a skipping rope with frayed rope may slip during your routine and cause injury.

It is also important that the equipment you use be rated in kilograms or pounds. When you use a weight that is too heavy for you, not only will it cause injuries but you will gain no benefit from your routine. On the other hand, if the weights are too light for you, it makes no sense wasting your time doing exercises with them.

Another area to remember is that of DIY home-exercising equipment. If you are considering making your own equipment, such as dumbbells or a homemade skipping rope, make sure you know what you're doing. If in doubt, purchase the equipment. Homemade weights can be dangerous if the size or weight rating is incorrect.

Another important issue to ensure safety is the location of the equipment. If you are using a bench or staider, make sure it is sturdy and that no one can trip over it. Make sure the area where you are exercising is free from obstructions such as carpets or rugs so that you don't lose your balance.

Another area of personal safety to think about is any other family members who may be present when you are exercising. For example, you may be using a bench or staider when someone else is also using it. Give them plenty of room to exercise and be careful not to trip over them. Also, make sure you get out of their way when they are coming towards you.

Secondly, consider any young children who may be present when you are exercising. It is a good idea to put them in front of the television or entertain them in another room to distract them from wanting to play around while you are exercising.

You should also be sure to have a cold drink handy to keep hydrated while you are exercising.

Lastly, if you have pets or pets visiting, be wary of them. Some pets may get scared by the exercises you are doing and run away or try to jump on you when you are using the equipment. If this is the case, find another room for exercising or create some barriers so your pet can't get to you without your knowledge.

Following those tips above, you can ensure a safe and comfortable environment for exercising at home.

## HOW TO MAKE SURE YOUR HOME EXERCISES ARE ALWAYS SAFE.

Working out at home is an excellent option for those who live in a climate where the weather prohibits outdoor activity, or those who otherwise lack the time to devote to a lengthy workout routine. There are many form of exercises that can be done inside your home, but it's important to remember that not all exercises are appropriate for every person. You may need someone with medical expertise to help determine which exercise you should start with and what modifications will be necessary in order to achieve your full range of motion and avoid potential injury.

In addition, some exercises may require modification to enable you to do them safely. For example, if your planks are causing pain in your wrists or elbows, they may be too challenging for you. It's also very important to remember that you should always consult your physician before beginning an exercise program.

When performing home exercises, it is important that you make sure that proper form is being used. If you lift weights from the wrong positions (e.g. lifting from the knees), you may cause severe injury to the muscles of the back, shoulders, or neck.

So to avoid this certain kind of problem make sure that your home exercises are always safe. The following will tell and guide you on how to make sure your home exercises are always safe:

1. Make sure you are physically fit. If you are inflexible, then normal exercises may not be safe for you.
2. Always consult your physician before starting an exercise program. Your physician should know the meaning of any medical terms used in your home exercise program, and should be able to help you identify any potential health concerns and make necessary modifications accordingly.
3. Consider consulting a fitness professional for advice before starting an exercise program at home.
4. Always consult your physician before starting an exercise program, and make sure to check your range of motion to know how much you can do without injuring yourself.
5. Be careful when working out in hot environments at your home.
6. Always train with a partner, especially if you are lifting weights, because this will help prevent injury during training.

7. Have proper posture. Poor posture can cause aches and pains throughout the body; poor upper-body posture can lead to shoulder pain, headaches, or shoulder blade pain.

8. Never train in a situation that you are unsure of. If you have no clue what you are doing, then it is best to ask an instructor or trainer for help with your particular exercise.

9. Learn proper exercise form and technique. If you don't know the proper position for an exercise, avoid making any sudden movements, especially if the movement is something that could damage or damage your body parts.

10. Use correct form when doing any movements that may lead to injury.

11. Always remember to warm up before you start an exercise program, and appropriately cool down afterward.

12. When doing any exercise, always remember to breathe properly.

13. Do not do any exercise if you are feeling dizzy or momentarily unable to breathe.

14. Always consult your physician before starting an exercise program for more specific advice concerning what exercises you can do safely at your home, and how much you can lift.

15. Do not strain yourself when doing your home exercises. If you are struggling with a specific exercise, do only as much as you can without straining. It is preferable to take precautions rather than risk injury by pushing yourself too hard.

16. Stop exercising if you feel any pain or discomfort in your joints or muscles during an exercise. Pain means that the muscle is being stressed, so stop immediately if you feel pain and examine the area for damage.

17. To properly cool down, you should perform a slow and gentle stretching after the end of a workout.

18. After your exercise program, always stretch and move slowly to help reduce your risk of any future injury.

Making sure your home exercises are always safe is important to help prevent injury while training. If you take the time to follow the listed safety tips, your home exercises will be safe, and you can be safe from any potential injuries that may occur while performing any exercise at your home. Remember that safety first is a must, and with the proper precautions, any of your home exercises can be safe, and may help you reach any fitness goals you may have.

# 7

# HOME EXERCISES FOR VARIOUS SPECIAL NEEDS

Everyone has their own special needs, so it makes sense to work out your body in a way that works best for you. Make sure to consult your doctor before beginning any new workout program.

When you exercise at home, find out what works best for you and stick with that. You can do exercises that are targeted to your problem areas or work on flexibility and core stability which will not only help alleviate pain, it will also reduce the chance of future injury.

Mobility issues can be caused by injuries, arthritis, spinal cord injuries, or other conditions. Your doctor might advise you to get physical therapist to prescribe exercises that will help improve the mobility of your body. The chosen exercises will depend on the area you are trying to improve. Exercises for your arm, hand, shoulder, leg and foot mobility can help improve your mobility. You can do these some exercises at home or work on them with a physical therapist to ensure you are doing them correctly.

Strengthening your lower back is another important step toward improving your mobility and reducing any pain you may be experiencing. You can do this by targeting the abs, glutes and lower back muscles.

Core stability is important for reducing back pain and improving overall function. You can do lunges, sit-ups, pull-ups and bicycle crunches to strengthen your core so that you can maintain proper spinal alignment during flexion and extension movements. Core stability exercises are important at home if you have an injury or condition.

Flexibility training is important for reducing back pain, improving the range of motion in your joints, decreasing muscle spasms and increasing blood circulation. You can use different flexibility exercises for each joint and also target different joints. Flexibility exercises can also be done at home to target specific joints.

Stretching should be part of your daily exercise routine if you have joint pain and low back discomfort in particular. These exercises will improve flexibility, reduce muscle tension, and help decrease pain during everyday movements.

## HOME EXERCISES FOR MULTIPLE SCLEROSIS, RHEUMATOID ARTHRITIS, PROSTATE PROBLEMS, TREATED BACK PAIN, AND RHEUMATIC DISEASES.

Multiple Sclerosis is a chronic immune-system disease that affects how the central nervous system communicates with the rest of the body. Symptoms can vary significantly from person to person, but often include muscle weakness, fatigue, loss of coordination or balance, numbness in parts of the body and changes in sensation such as hot or cold sensations. In addition to physical symptoms, MS patients may also experience depression and anxiety.

Rheumatoid Arthritis is a chronic inflammatory disease that can affect the ends of the bones in your wrists, knees, ankles, fingers and shoulders. The disease causes a number of painful symptoms, including stiffness, pain and swelling in the joints. Over time, these symptoms can cause your joints to lose their shape and mobility.

Prostate Problems is common among men who have high-risk prostate cancer. Prostate Problems can be a symptom of prostate cancer or it may be a separate condition. Prostate problems can involve the urinary tract and can cause men to urinate more often or more urgently, in addition to frequent urination during the night. As a result of frequent urination, men may also experience incontinence, or unintentional loss of bladder control.

Treated Back Pain is a typical condition for people who have suffered from back pain on and off for years, but there are also many other possible causes. Back pain can be a symptom of a serious condition such as a spinal injury, arthritis or a herniated disk. It can also result from overuse of your back, such as with repetitive motion injuries or lifting heavy objects.

Rheumatic Diseases is a broad category of disorders that affect the joints, muscles and connective tissue. Overlapping with other categories of autoimmune disorders, rheumatic diseases include arthritis, lupus and fibromyalgia. It can cause the joints in the body to become inflamed, and cause intense pain. Rheumatic diseases can cause swelling, stiffness, and pain in the joints of the body.

Exercise is not just for getting in shape - it's a natural way to heal from disease. Along with the proper diet for your condition, exercise can help reduce inflammation and make life easier with less pain.

This will show you some simple and effective home exercises that are good for many chronic conditions including Multiple Sclerosis, Rheumatoid Arthritis, Prostate Problems, Treated Back Pain, and Rheumatic Diseases.

1. Stretching is an important part of any exercise program. You can stretch out your muscles before or after you work out, or both. Stretching also helps prevent soreness and injury.
2. Begin by standing for at least 5 minutes and take a few deep breaths to relax yourself before you begin a Kegel exercise

routine or any physical activity that may cause muscle fatigue or soreness.

3. Strengthen your legs by lying on your back and slowly lifting one leg up from the bottom, while keeping your torso on the floor. You can also do a Leg Lift with both legs at once (a V-sit). This is a great exercise to strengthen your hips and core.

4. Hold the v-sit for as long as possible while breathing normally. If you feel dizzy or lightheaded, then stop.

5. Exercise your arms by holding onto a sturdy chair seat, and lift one arm out straight from your shoulder and hold for a few seconds and then switch arms. This is also good for stretching out your core muscles in your abdomen. You will probably have to hold on with one hand at first while you get used to the exercise and build up some strength.

6. Hold a plank position (where you hold your body in a straight line from head to toe and maintain that position) for as long as you can while breathing normally.

7. Walk around the house for 5 minutes while doing some light stretches.

8. Stretch out your lower back by sitting on the floor and reaching behind you to grasp your legs or hold onto a sturdy chair seat.

9. Exercise your core muscles (abs, hip flexors, and lower back) by lying down on the floor and lifting your legs up against a wall. Do at least 5 repetitions.

10. With your back lying on the floor, prop your legs up on a wall or sturdy chair and try to lift your torso up off the floor while holding onto something.

11. Stretch your lower back further by leaning over and holding onto a chair or table with one hand while reaching for your other foot with the other to touch it.

Exercising regularly reduces fatigue and improves overall sleep in patients with multiple sclerosis, rheumatoid arthritis, or treated back pain. Regular exercise also helped those with prostate problems and rheumatic diseases patients cope better with the disease. These simple tips will help you how to exercise at home and help treat conditions like Multiple Sclerosis, Rheumatoid Arthritis, Prostate Problems, Treated Back Pain, and Rheumatic Diseases.

## AN OVERVIEW OF HOME EXERCISES FOR ARTHRITIS.

We all know that to stay healthy, we have to exercise. This is especially true for people who suffer from arthritis. The joints in the body are susceptible to degeneration and it's not uncommon for them to be inflamed or even shattered by the time one reaches old age. Exercise increases blood flow, helps keep weight down, and builds muscle strength which decreases pressure on the joints — all important things when living with arthritis.

### 1. Joint mobilization.

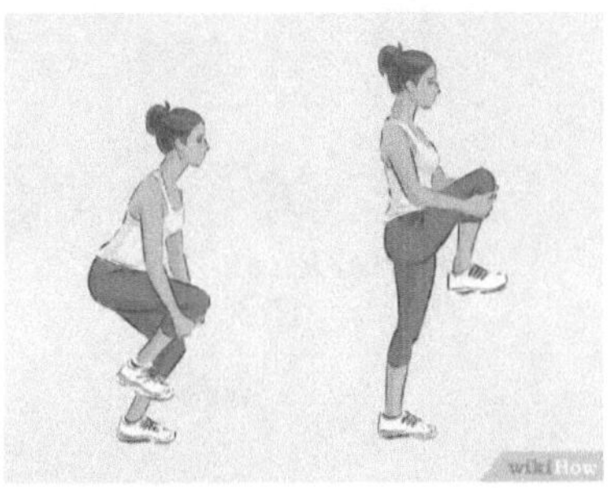


This is effective in reducing arthritis pain, increasing joint mobility, and improving muscle strength. Assume the position of the "seated cobra" and use your arms to lift your knees high off the floor so that you're balancing on your knees with only your toes touching the floor (this is called standing on tiptoe). Hold for 10-15 seconds, and then relax and repeat.

## 2. Wall push-ups.

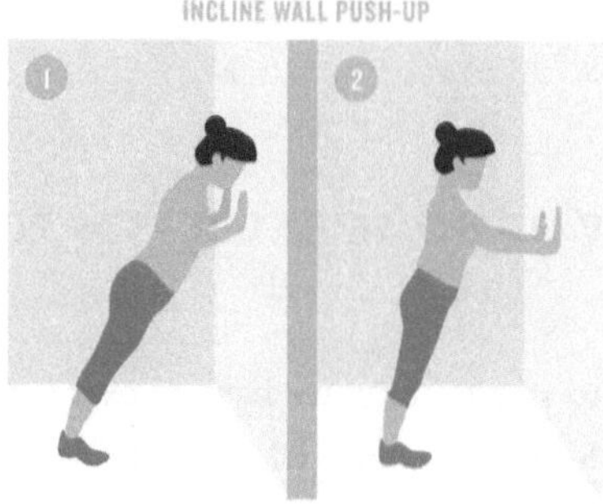


Stand against a wall with your feet shoulder-width apart. Lean forward and place both hands on the wall about six inches from your shoulder. Straighten your arms, keeping your body straight. Slowly slide down the wall until your chest touches the ground. Hold for 10-15 seconds, then raise back up to the starting position. Do five sets of ten reps, with a one-minute rest between sets.

## 3. Wall squats.

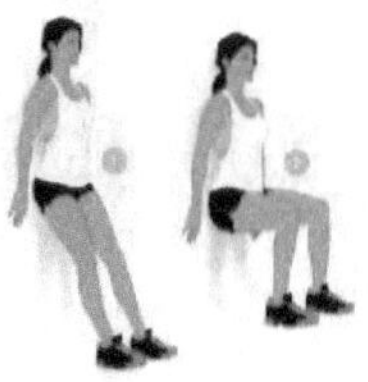

Stand with your feet shoulder-width apart and place both hands behind your head with fingers interlocked. Slowly bend both knees and slide down the wall until both knees are bent at a 90-degree angle. Hold for 10-15 seconds, then raise back up to the starting position. Do five sets of ten reps, with a one-minute rest between sets.

## 4. Wall pushups, heels on the floor.

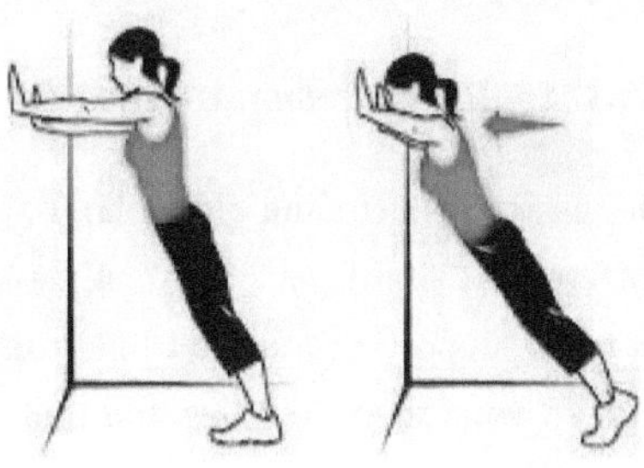

Stand in the same position as wall pushups and place your heels on the floor so that your legs are fully extended, with toes still touching the wall. Straighten your arms, keeping your body straight. Slowly slide down the wall until your chest touches the ground. Hold for 10-15 seconds, then raise back up to the starting position. Do five sets of ten reps, with a one-minute rest between sets.

## 5. Seated rows with an elastic resistance band.

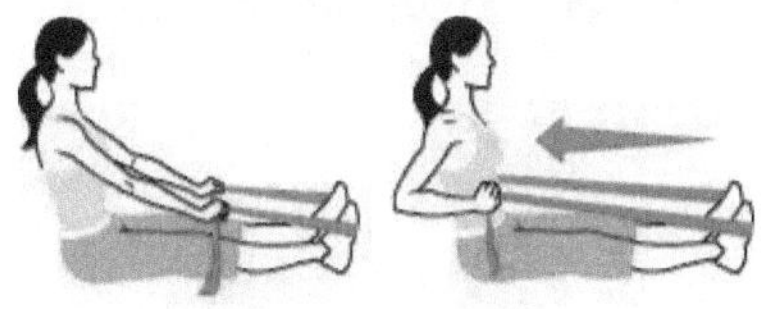

Sit on a chair and loop an elastic resistance band around a leg of the chair at knee level so that you have two handles in front of you. Holding both handles, lean forward from the hips and pull your elbow toward your knee. Hold for 10-15 seconds, then release. Do five sets of ten reps, with a one-minute rest between sets.

## 6. Bicep curls with an elastic resistance band.

Sit on a chair with both knees bent and place one foot on the floor near the chair to support you (at shin level). Loop an elastic resistance band around the ankle of the supporting foot and hold the other end in one hand. Slowly straighten your supporting leg and pull your hand toward shoulder height, bending your elbow. Hold for 10-15 seconds, then release. Do five sets of ten reps, with a one-minute rest between sets.

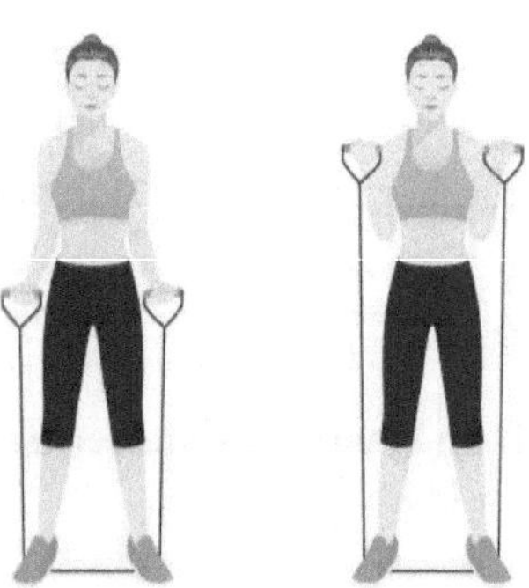

## 7. Seated chest press with an elastic resistance band.

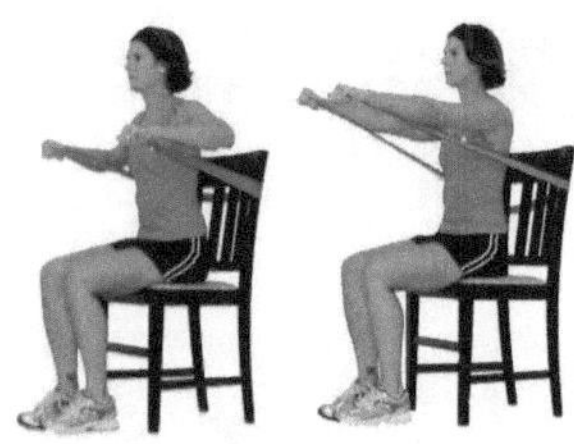

Sit on a chair and loop an elastic resistance band around both legs just above the knees so that you have one handle in each hand. Hold the handles in front of you with your arms extended and elbows locked. Slowly press the handles together, keeping your elbows locked. Hold for 10-15 seconds, then release. Do five sets of ten reps, with a one-minute rest between sets.

## 8. Leg lifts in a chair.

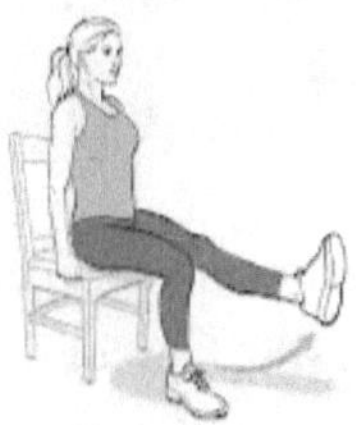

Sit on a chair or bench with your knees bent at 90-degree angles and hold both hands behind your head (fingers interlocked). Use your arms to lift your legs high off the ground so that both knees are straight. Hold for 10-15 seconds, and then relax and repeat. Do five sets of ten reps, with a one-minute rest between sets.

## 9. Heel lifts in a chair with an elastic resistance band.

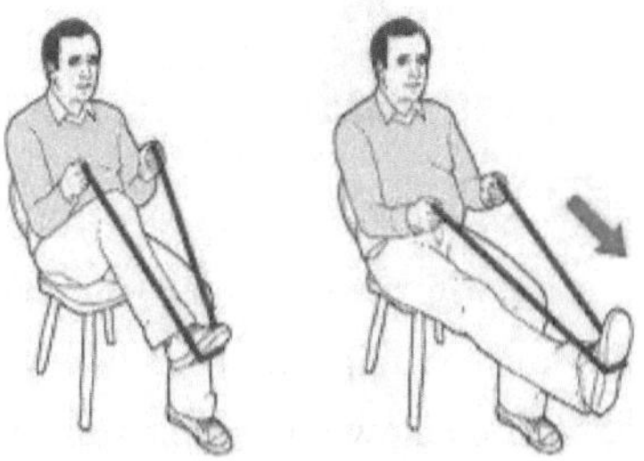

Sit on a chair and loop an elastic resistance band around one leg, at shin level, so that you have both handles in one hand. Place both hands on the front edge of the seat and straighten your supporting leg so that it is bent at a right angle. Hold for 10-15 seconds, then release. Do five sets of ten reps, with a one-minute rest between sets.

## 10. The standing calf raise.

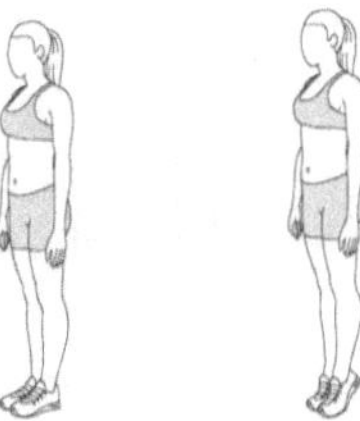

Stand facing a wall with the toes of your right foot touching the wall for balance. Place both hands on your hips for support. Raise up onto the ball of your left foot and hold for 10-15 seconds, then relax and repeat. Do five sets of ten reps, with a one-minute rest between sets.

## 11. Supine leg raises.

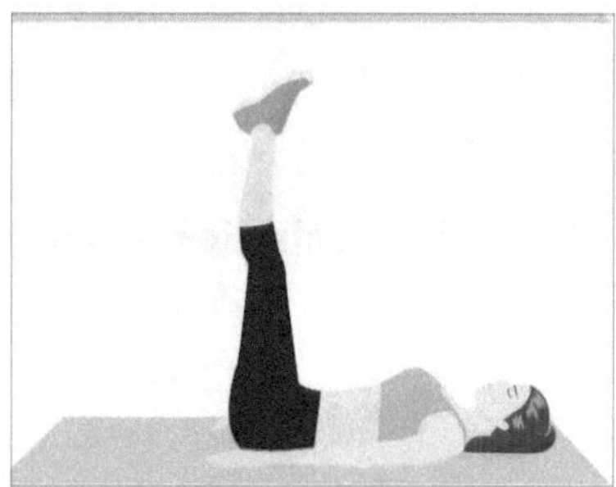

Lay face down and place your hands under your forehead with elbows extended and palms down. Straighten your legs while simultaneously extending both arms at the elbow (and pulling them toward you). Hold for 10-15 seconds, and then relax and repeat. Do five sets of ten reps, with a one-minute rest between sets.

## 12. Side lying leg lifts with an elastic resistance band.

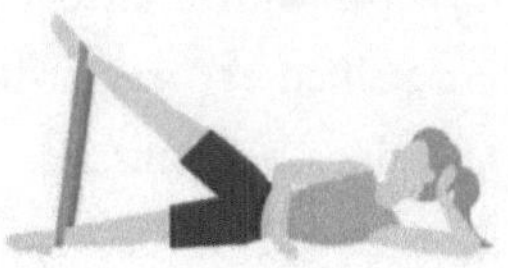

Sit at the edge of a chair and loop an elastic resistance band around one leg, at shin level. Hold the both handles in front of you with your arms extended and elbows locked. Slowly bend your supporting leg and lift it up to the side of your body while simultaneously pulling the elastic band toward you with both hands. Hold for 10-15 seconds, then release. Do five sets of ten reps, with a one-minute rest between sets.

## 13. Side lying triceps extensions with an elastic resistance band.

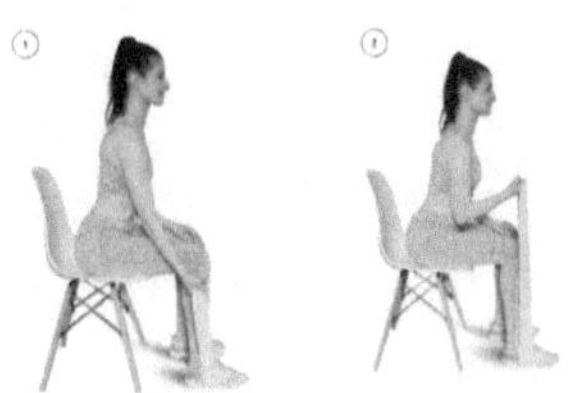

Sit on a chair and loop an elastic resistance band around one foot, just below the ankle. Hold one handle in each hand and lean back so that your body is at a 45-degree angle. Straighten your supporting arm and pull the elastic band toward you, extending your elbow. Hold for 10-15 seconds, then release. Do five sets of ten reps, with a one-minute rest between sets.

These home exercises are proven to have a great impact on people having arthritis, but also benefit people with a knee injury or surgery. Since many of the exercises are classified as "weight-bearing," they will help strengthen your ligaments, tendons, and muscles.

8

# HOME EXERCISES FOR WEIGHT LOSS

Weight loss exercises are an essential component to weight loss. Your muscles will burn more fat than your stomach can while at rest, and strength training is proven to have a significant effect on how quickly your body burns calories. Exercise also helps the body fight off disease, strengthens bones and joints, improves blood flow, reduces stress levels and even increases energy levels.

Active people who are overweight report feeling better, sleeping better, and even looking better than those who are not fit. Regular exercise can also protect against injury and reduce the risk of diabetes, high blood pressure, and heart disease.

It's important to note that a healthy diet and regular physical activity are two key components that make up a weight loss program. If you try to lose weight without making these habits a priority, your efforts can easily backfire. Of course this is not the only component to consider; some people require more exercise than others in order for them to reach their ideal weight. By way of example, a person of moderately active would be considered overweight while someone who is very physically active would be considered obese. This is simply a factor of body fat percentages. While exercise can help you lose weight, it shouldn't be the only component to your weight loss program.

Weight Loss Exercises are important because they burn calories and increase muscle mass. On average, physical activity burns calories at the rate of 3-5 calories per 1 pound of muscle per day. This implies that the more muscle you have, the more calories you burn. The 20 minute difference between your aerobic and strength training workout has been shown to result in a difference of roughly 400 calories over the day.

So why is weight loss exercise so important? To understand, consider that fat is metabolically active tissue. As a result of this, a person's weight can cause metabolic health problems such as increased blood glucose or cholesterol levels. If you want to optimize your body's ability to handle these problems, then you need to make sure that there are no additional health issues that are currently affecting it. In this way, weight loss exercise can help prevent future cardiovascular health issues and improve your overall metabolic health.

## HOME EXERCISES FOR WEIGHT LOSS, INCLUDING DIET AND EXERCISE.

Being overweight is not always an indicator of your health. If you are overweight but maintaining good blood pressure, no history of heart disease or diabetes and not experiencing any joint pain, then it is likely that your weight is healthy and within a normal range. But if you are overweight and your blood pressure is on the higher side, you have a history of heart disease or diabetes or you're experiencing joint pain then it is high time that you do something about it.

*What is the best way to lose weight?*

The best way to lose weight is through diet, exercise and taking weight loss supplements. If the diet and exercise part seems too much for you then take help from a good weight loss supplement. But if you want to lose weight in a more natural way then try these home exercises for weight loss, including diet and exercise.

Is the home exercise method effective?

Yes, it is. There such a number of studies that have proved that home exercises for weight loss and dieting are an effective way of shedding pounds. The result you get is not only good but also faster than the other methods of weight loss. As and when you lose weight, you will become healthier and more active.

*What kind of exercises should I do to lose weight the right way?*

To lose weight in a healthy way try to do cardiovascular exercises like jogging, brisk walking, aerobics and the like. You can also rev up your metabolism by doing weights exercises or resistance exercise. Resistance exercises help tone your muscles giving you that fit body that you desire.

Home Exercises for Weight Loss, including diet and exercise:

## 1. Cardiovascular Exercises:

Cardiovascular exercises are vital to lose weight. They help you burn off more calories than other exercises and also helps you lose weight faster. The best thing about cardiovascular exercises is that they can be done almost anywhere and anytime.

*How to do it:*

To tone up your heart into a shape of a lean machine, try doing cardio-vascular exercise every day for at least 30 minutes or even an hour daily. You don't have to do your exercises all at one time either. You can break it up into smaller sessions every day. If you are short of time then try doing interval training instead of long and continuous workouts. The interval training will not only reduce the time you spend on your workouts but will also burn more calories than those for long and continuous workouts.

## 2. Resistance Exercises:

Resistance training with weights is a much better way of burning off excess calories than other exercises. It helps tone up your muscles, helps you build those lean muscles and also reduces the fat in your body without making you feel tired or exhausted. Resistance training also teaches your muscles how to function better, enabling them to burn more calories even while at rest.

*How to do it:*

Resistance involves using weights, springs or cables to exercise the different resistance bands of muscle groups in your body. The best thing about resistance training is that it is effective at burning calories even during rest. You can do this as often as you want, as long as you have the time and energy to spare.

## 3. Home Exercise Program:

A home exercise program is a great way of losing weight. It brings all the exercises listed above together into one weight loss plan that does not require a gym membership or other membership fees. It is also very easy to carry out. All you need to do is prepare a list of exercises from this list and keep repeating them from day to day.

*How to do it:*

For a start, choose any of the above exercise and carry it out daily for at least 10 minutes or as recommended by your doctor/trainer. The target time can be increased gradually with time. Once you can do each of the exercises for a set time, try doing them in 1-minute intervals. If possible, start with just 1 minute at a time and build up slowly.

Each day, add another exercise to the list and repeat the steps for that exercise again. Follow these steps one after the other until you have completed all of them. The exercises listed above have already been tried and tested by many people and are quite effective in losing weight without making you feel tired or fatigued.

## 4. Weight Loss Supplements:

Weight loss supplements are an excellent way of shedding excess pounds and toning your muscles at the same time. They help burn fat as well as boost the metabolism, helping you lose weight in no time at all. All you need to do is follow a weight loss supplement plan and you will see results.

Weight loss supplements can be purchased by anyone over 18 years of age and this does not mean that they are not effective or safe. They are quite safe but it is important to follow the instructions given on the bottle and do not take more than recommended. Regular use of weight loss supplements ensure that you achieve your weight loss goals without making necessary changes in your lifestyle.

## 5. Yoga for Weight Loss:

Yoga is an ancient Indian technique that helps you balance your mind and body. It has existed for a very long time and can be used to lose weight, maintain a good body shape as well as promote overall health. It is a great exercise method to aid your weight loss goals and also keep you from feeling tired or exhausted after a workout. However, like all other exercises it is important to do yoga under the guidance of a good trainer or yoga teacher in order to get the desired results.

## 6. Aerobics:

Aerobics are a great way of shedding unwanted pounds and toning your body. They are basically a series of exercises that involve moving the body in various motions. Choose any aerobics program and it will help you shed excess pounds and also help tone your body muscles. You can choose from a variety of aerobics programs to meet your requirements and taste.

## 7. Tai Chi:

Tai Chi is a great way to bring balance and harmony into your life. It helps strengthen your body and mind while improving circulation and mental clarity. It also reduces stress levels, increases energy levels, improves cardiovascular health as well as helps you lose weight. With the right Tai Chi program, you can lose weight quite fast while feeling good about yourself at the same time.

Remember that home exercises for weight loss, including diet and exercise are highly recommended by doctors and trainers. Remember to always consult your doctor before trying out any form of exercise and avoid using weight loss pills without a doctor's approval.

Most of these exercises are easy to follow and don't require any special training or gym equipment for you to get the desired results. Always start light initially before you try out tougher exercises as a way of maintaining good body health.

## HOW TO LOSE WEIGHT WITH HOME EXERCISES.

Losing weight doesn't have to be difficult. There are actually lot of effective ways to slim down, and the simplest is just by doing a few home exercises each day for a few minutes.

It is possible to be really fit and healthy without ever having to step foot inside a gym! When you do have home exercises, you are saving yourself both time and money because you can get fit in the comfort of your own home.

In fact, home exercises can be even more effective than going to the gym because you have the liberty to do them whenever or wherever you want. With home exercises, there is no need to plan hours in advance just to squeeze in a workout.

## How to lose weight with home exercises:

### 1. Do sit-ups at home.

Sit-ups work out the abdominal muscles, which helps tone the chest and arms. It also strengthens the back and shoulders, making it easier to carry heavy loads such as grocery bags.

How to do this: Lie on your back and place your hands behind your head or cross your hands at the middle of the chest. Align your elbows with your shoulders. Lift your chest and then tuck in your chin.

### 2. Do crunches at home.

Crunches work out the stomach muscles, which are important for looking slimmer and maintaining a healthy shape of the abdomen. Crunches also work out the back muscles and this helps improve posture so that you will not hunch over when stressed.

How to do this: Lie on your back and place your hands behind your head or cross your hands at the middle of the chest. Align your elbows with your shoulders. Lift your torso and tuck in your chin.

### 3. Do push-ups at home.

Push-ups work out the chest area, making you look slimmer and sexier.

How to do: Place both feet on the floor or rest one foot on a flat stool while keeping the other foot firmly planted on the floor. Hold your body in a straight line from shoulders to knees. Keep your head up and look forward.

### 4. Do bicep curls at home.

Bicep curls exercises are also done at home and help strengthen the upper arm, which is important for reaching for objects or carrying heavy items, such as groceries or laundry baskets. This also helps reduce the appearance of flabby upper arms. It is amazing how this simple exercise can help you lose weight.

How to do: Stand on a step stool so that the balls of your toes touch the ground while still holding onto a bar attached to the step stool. Alternatively, have someone hold you at the waist and lift your feet a few inches off the ground. Hold your arms straight out while lifting the weight.

### 5. Do shoulder shrugs at home.

Shoulder shrugs help strengthen the upper arm, which is important for lifting heavy objects or carrying them for a long distance. This also helps reduce the appearance of flabby upper arms.

How to do: Stand up straight and look straight ahead. With both shoulders shrugged, bend at the elbows to one side so that your right elbow hugs your left upper arm. Clasp your hands behind your back or in front of you as if you were about to pray. Slowly return from the starting position without locking out at the top or dropping down to the floor.

### 6. Do arm circles at home.

Arm circles help tone the forearms and wrists, which are important for reaching objects or carrying them for a long distance. This is also an excellent way to burn calories throughout the day because you can do it whenever you want.

How to do: Stand flat-footed with your arms at your sides. While keeping your shoulders down and back straight, turn your arms inward at the elbow in one continuous motion while keeping one palm facing forward.

### 7. Do pull-ups at home.

Pull-ups are the best exercise to tone the back and biceps. This exercise is one of the most effective ways to burn fat in the back. It could also help in the reduction of cellulite appearance, which can be added to your lower arms and thighs.

How to do: Start by grabbing on to a bar attached to a high ceiling or building. Pull yourself up using your arms and abs so that you're in an inverted position with your head at eye level and shoulders down. Press your feet against the ground in a push-up position.

*8. Do squats at home.*

Squats help tone the thighs, making it easier to carry heavy items for a long distance. It also works out the knees, making them more flexible and less likely to give out on you while carrying or walking through the house. Squats also work out the buttocks, which is important when you sit down on an object for a long time for example driving or watching television.

How to do this: Stand up straight with your feet together. Make sure that both your heels and the toes are touching the ground. Look straight ahead, keep your hands at a normal distance from the body or behind the head like a soldier. Slowly bend down until the legs are at a right angle and then back up again. Inhale if you go down and exhale when you go up.

*9. Do wall push-ups at home.*

Wall push-ups help strengthen the upper arms and chest muscles without having to do conventional or regular push-ups. Wall push-ups are also a good way to lose weight because they help tone the upper arm muscles.

How to do: Stand up straight and look straight ahead. Place your forearms on a wall with elbows bent. Slowly lean forward so that your body, elbows and forearms are horizontal to the ground. Your palms should be facing down, not facing each other or backwards. Slowly return to the starting position without locking your elbows at the top or dropping down to the floor.

*10. Do sit-ups with a twist at home.*

Sit-ups with a twist help tone your upper back, if it is not excessive. This exercise is also effective for toning the chest muscles and helps reduce the appearance of flabby chest.

How to do: Lie on your back and place one arm above your head while keeping the other arm outstretched by your side. Align your elbows with your shoulders. Lift your torso and tuck in your chin. At the same time, rotate the opposite side of your body to bring it toward the upper arm that is above you -while keeping your head up and looking forward.

With these exercises, a beautiful and slimmer body is yours for the taking! For the best results, try these at least 2-3 times a week for 30-60 seconds each, keeping your calories in check. Remember that you can always work out at home as part of your routine every day.

# 9

# HOW TO GET THE RIGHT EQUIPMENT TO IMPROVE YOUR HOME EXERCISES

## CHOOSING THE RIGHT HOME EXERCISE EQUIPMENT FOR YOU.

Exercise equipment is available in a variety of different types, and they all serve a specific purpose.

Some equipment is designed for general use, whereas others are designed for one particular activity or sport.

If you're looking to start doing some exercise at home, then it's important to choose the right type of equipment so that you can make the most of your time. It's also important to choose an exercise routine that works best for you and fits into your busy schedule.

With the right equipment, you can get whatever exercise you desire at home. You can do so without purchasing unnecessary luxury items or breaking the bank. However, it's important to choose the right equipment based on your current fitness level and needs. Here are some tips for choosing home exercise equipment.

Consider how often you want to exercise. If you only want to do it once a month, then look for a piece of equipment that doesn't take up much room. You can also get a treadmill that folds down into your home's walkway and tracks your progress.

Consider if you have space in your home for the exercise equipment. Not all exercises need to have the same amount of space, so pay attention to the size of an item when determining if it's right for you.

Do you need to use a lot of space for your exercise? If so, then a home gym is the way to go. You can get equipment that is designed specifically for the activities you want to perform at home.

Check how much it costs to purchase and maintain the equipment you choose. Some exercise equipment requires monthly payments in addition to a large initial price tag. It might not fit into your budget if it's not something you can afford every single month.

Do you want to do a variety of activities? If you're looking for equipment that helps you to do many different activities, then remember that it might require more maintenance.

Is it cost effective? Think about how many times you're willing to use the equipment before throwing it away. If it's not something that will last long, then again, choose something else. In addition, think about where the equipment is made and consider what materials are used in the construction of the equipment.

Review the warranty. Make sure to read the warranty before choosing exercise equipment. It might not be worth it if you can't get a replacement quickly if it breaks down.

So, you can see that there are many things to consider when choosing home exercise equipment. If you want to get fit at home, then make sure that you choose something that will work for your needs and budget. Remember to choose an appropriate machine based on your own fitness level and needs so that you can make the most out of your time at home.

## HOME EXERCISE EQUIPMENT

The use of exercise equipment at home can help people get fit in ways that are beneficial to their health and well-being. Research on fitness has shown this to be true. In order for a person, or an entire group, to get results, it is important that they apply the same level of commitment and discipline as in the gym. There are many different types of equipment today.

Here are some types of equipment:

**Weight-Resistance devices** range from free weights to machines that have free weights and flywheels or cables. Users can choose the resistance of the weight based on their strength and physical condition. Weight-resistance machines include dumbbells, barbells, power racks, and hexagonal bars or other shapes. The beauty of weight-resistance equipment is that users can adjust the amount of resistance by adding more weights or lowering them to compensate for strength changes brought on by injury or normal aging. Weight-resistance devices may also be used for calisthenics, or exercises that use only the weight of one's body to perform the movements.

**Funmats and other foam mats** on the floor provide a soft surface for exercising virtually anywhere. These mats provide both strength and flexibility components, by combining cycles of standing on and off (similar to Pilates) with single-leg lifts, squats, pushups, pull-ups, skullshishes, crunches and upper-body workouts using bands, pulleys and other equipment.

**Dumbbells and barbells** are used to add resistance to muscles by increasing the resistance on the weight one is lifting. Dumbbells, also known as free weights, are weights smaller than barbells and are usually made of metal or rubber. Barbells include iron plates of varying lengths or diameter used for lifting heavy weights. These plates are designed for strict adherence to the international Weightlifting Federation rules of lifting that stipulate how much weight a lifter can lift.

**Resistance bands** consist of flat, thick strips of rubber or plastic that range in length from one to eighty or more feet used for strength training and stretching. These are usually not as restrictive on the joints as weight machines because they are not bolted. There is no preset resistance, so users can vary the amount of resistance by changing how tight they pull on the band. Resistance bands can be used for a variety of exercises that combine different muscle groups.

**Exercise balls** are available in sizes suitable for children, multiple sports, and adults. They can be used for a variety of exercises that increase strength in the arms, abdomen muscles and back. These types of equipment can be used indoors or outdoors.

**Stair machines** may help with cardiovascular exercise and burns calories by raising the heart rate quickly. Stair machines can help strengthen the muscles of the upper and lower body, especially if used at full resistance.

**Trampolines** are usually round or oval shaped and may be one to three inches thick. They provide cardiovascular exercise, due to the rapid movements of rebounding up and down from a trampoline. Trampolines also provide a good aerobic workout for those with arthritis because they also involve movement of all joints.

# 10

# THE RIGHT MINDSET FOR YOUR HOME EXERCISES

## THE IMPORTANCE OF HAVING THE RIGHT MINDSET BEFORE STARTING HOME EXERCISES.

Before beginning a workout routine the most important things you can do is having a positive mindset and attitude about it. Having the right mindset before starting any exercise is crucial because it puts you in a mentally positive state of mind and makes you want to do the exercises.

Having the right mindset can be a motivational tool to have when you are performing home exercises. The best way to make yourself want to do the exercises is to have a good attitude towards them. If you see the exercises as a chore, it will be very easy for you not to complete them. Instead of seeing the exercises as a chore, see them as something that you want to achieve or need. Remember that not all exercises are easy, so it might be hard at times to do them. You eventually have to pull through the exercises and see them as something you want to achieve. It is a lot easier for your body to exercise if you know what you are training for. Think about being in a race and wanting to do well or being in a football game and wanting it more than your opponent. Being in a good mindset can also help you with this by motivating your ability to do the exercises at hand.

Another importance of having a good mindset is to see yourself as an athlete. When you see yourself as an athlete, your attention gets directed to your movements and you are motivated that there is something you want to achieve through the exercises. The best way to achieve this mindset is by visualizing what you want or what you are training for at the time of exercise. Visualization makes you feel like you are training for something and that can increase your motivation in performing exercises.

The right mindset is crucial for a good workout. If you are in a bad mood during home exercises or having any other negative feelings, the likelihood of you following through with the exercises is very slim. The best way to have a positive mood while working out is to do it with your friends. When you are doing home workouts with your friends, there is more motivation to continue because they will not let you give up easily. Keeping yourself company while doing workouts can be fun and can create a good mood for exercising more. Not only is having friends around more fun but it promotes a positive atmosphere for working out.

Having the proper mindset allows you to keep a positive attitude while doing home exercises. Having good results from the exercises is based on your motivation to do it. The biggest thing that holds people back from exercising is the fact that they do not have a very motivated or good mindset when they start. If you are not in a bad mood and are not feeling lazy, you will be more likely to continue exercising than if you are in a negative state. If you want to get a good workout, be positive about the exercises and do them with an open mind.

In order to keep yourself motivated while exercising, it is important to try and maintain your motivation over time. Once you feel bored with the exercises or thoughts come into your head that makes it difficult for you to exercise, this can cause your motivation for exercising to decrease over time. Always keep your motivation up by constantly motivating yourself.

Motivation can be maintained by trying new workouts that you are interested in.

## HOW TO MAKE SURE YOUR HOME EXERCISES ARE SUCCESSFUL, EVEN WHEN YOU'RE UNDER A LOT OF STRESS.

We all know how hard it can be to fit in a workout when we're busy. After all, it's tough enough to find the time for working out when we aren't stressed or overwhelmed. But in reality, the more stress we're under, the more important it is to make sure we're exercising. A recent study found that a moderate level of stress can actually improve physical performance and mental well-being. But too much stress can also be bad for your health and can affect how you feel about exercise. So how exactly is stress related to our workouts? Stress hormones rise when we are faced with even minor amounts of pressure. These hormones, such as cortisol, adrenaline (epinephrine) and human growth hormone (GH), can help us meet the demands of a stressful situation. But experiencing too much stress or chronic stress can lead to problems like anxiety and depression. It can also hurt your health—increasing levels of cholesterol and causing some changes in the heart that are associated with high blood pressure. And it can affect how we feel about exercise. When we're experiencing a lot of stress, most people tend to lose interest in exercise.

Here are some steps that can help you stick with your home workout routine despite stress:

1. Make yourself accountable to someone else. For example, make a fitness member of your household or a friend do the same number of pushups as you do every day. This will give you a reason to keep up with the workout routine and help you avoid feeling isolated and discouraged.
2. Find an alternative way to deal with stress while you are exercising. Many people find it helpful to exercise while

listening to music or meditating. The choices are limitless here, so pick something that works for you!

3. Don't get discouraged at the beginning. It may took 30 days for a new routine to become a part of your regular life. So don't just expect to feel like you love it from day one!

4. Don't push yourself too hard too soon. That can also lead to increased stress levels and more problems with sticking with the routine. Instead, gradually increase movement and the number of repetitions you do. Also, if you are new to exercising, you may find that working out on a regular basis is not enjoyable until your muscles get stronger. It's best to start with exercise that uses your whole body for a sustained period of time. You can also choose exercises that require lighter weights or more repetitions.

5. Keep track of how you feel. Pay attention to how you feel about exercise and your regular routine, and write them down every day. The more you know about your moods, the better you will be able to adjust your routine to the demands of your particular situation or stress level.

6. Choose activities that are fun and won't make you stressed out too much during exercise. A great idea is to visit a gym where you can try out new things. Or if you are trying to do some activities at home, pick something that you don't need a whole lot of equipment for. For example, tai chi or yoga are both great options that are easy to do and don't require too much space or time.

7. Change it up! Sometimes altering the routine is the best way to stay interested and motivated. A good way to do this is to try something new every once in a while. You can even switch days and go for a walk on a different day of the week.

8. Deal with stress in other ways that don't involve exercise. You might carry some stress at work or at home, but you'll be able to avoid letting it take over your life if you find other ways to deal

with it. For example, make sure to talk to your doctor about any problems you have and find ways of coping with stress at home.

9.  Talk to someone about your frustrations and feelings about exercising. Talking to a friend or therapist can help you let go of negative emotions related to exercise and give you some good ideas on how exactly you should be dealing with stress.

10. Exercise with others. If there is someone in your family member who are interested in trying a fitness routine, or if there is a gym at your work that you can be part of, walk or exercise with friends. That way even if you don't feel like it, you are half tempted to go! Try and make sure that you have fun during exercise, so that your stress doesn't linger.

# 11

# HOW TO START DOING YOUR HOME EXERCISES TODAY

## THE TOP 10 TIPS FOR STARTING A HOME EXERCISE PROGRAM IN YOUR HOME.

Home exercise program is a great way to keep fit and stay motivated. If you have the motivation, this section will show you how to start your own home exercise program in your home with top 10 tips.

**#1. Find a workout buddy:** If you need someone else to push you in a workout, it is always best to find somebody who shares the same goal as yours and has similar fitness level with yours. Exercise can be much more enjoyable when there is somebody who also wants to achieve the same goals that we do. Not only that, having a workout partner can also help you to avoid the excuses of missing a workout.

**#2. Plan a schedule:** Having a schedule is much better than just doing random exercises and workouts. A proper plan will help you to stay on track and achieve your goal in fitness. Having a plan is also helpful in logging your progress and reviewing your program's effectiveness throughout the time. Here is the sample of a home exercise program schedule:

*A. Warm-up:* 5 minutes light jogging, skipping and light jogging (for beginners).

*B. Main workout:* 20 minutes of moderate intensity continuous workout like biking or rowing machine (It is best to buy an exercise machine with set timers). The intensity should be moderate as well as the time duration. Avoid high intensity workouts such as sprints or running for longer times than 20 minutes.

*C. Cool Down:* 5 minutes of light jogging (for beginners). Do not forget to stretch for your lower body and keep your heart rate low after the workout session.

It is very important for a beginner to master the warm-up and cool down exercises first before starting on their actual workout. It is also important to plan a workout schedule that will fit into your daily routine without being too intense.

**#3. Find the right workout equipment:** Exercise equipment is something that will make your workout program more enjoyable. No matter what kind of exercise you are doing, you will need to have a good pair of shoes to protect your feet. Other useful equipment includes weight lifting gloves, wrist wraps (for weight lifting), jump ropes and heart rate monitors. You can buy all the equipment that are needed in a home gym or simply buy an exercise machine which is suitable for your specific needs.

**#4. Find a workout space:** A good workout space in your home is very essential for an enjoyable workout program. For most people, a home gym will be the best option because it allows them to train individually and with more relaxation. But even without a home gym, there are plenty of possible solutions for training at home such as using stairs instead of an exercise machine or using the floor instead of a bench press machine.

**#5. Find a comfortable workout outfit:** There is no need to wear any fancy or colorful workout clothing to your home workouts. Above all, comfort should be the key point in choosing your workout clothes.

**#6 Buy some healthy snacks:** A good diet for an effective exercise session is very important. After all, your body will need plenty of energy to be able to perform well in daily workouts. You can buy healthy snacks such as fruit, vegetables and protein bars from grocery stores and convenience stores. Drink plenty of water during the workout session. Water can help you to stay hydrated as well as help you to prevent muscle pain and cramps.

**#7 Have patience:** Patience is one of the most important aspects in successful home exercise program. If you start off with intense workouts that are not suitable for your fitness level, you may end up hurting yourself instead of becoming fitter. If you feel that your program isn't working for you, take a good break and come back to it later until you have mastered it.

**#8 Make sure to keep your program flexible:** A flexible exercise routine will help you to adjust your workouts according to your needs and abilities. You may sometimes find out that a certain exercise is too difficult for you or not challenging enough. In this case, it is best to change workout schedule with something else instead of pushing yourself too hard just because there is nothing in the plan for today.

**#9 Remember that it takes time and effort to be fit:** It is not something that happens overnight. Even fitness experts cannot expect instant results from exercise workouts. It will take some changes in lifestyle and your diet as well as regular workouts to build a solid foundation for exercising regularly.

**#10 Keep it up:** This is the most important part of having a successful home exercise program. Even if you cannot do 100 push-ups in one go, you can still achieve great results by exercising regularly. If you want to lose weight, work out hard every day. If you want to build muscle mass, work out fast and intensely.

A home exercise program is important for a healthy and fit lifestyle. It does not matter if you are an expert or a beginner, as long as you are willing to put in the effort and enthusiasm into your fitness program, you will achieve great results.

All of the above are top 10 points that are important aspects to take into consideration when you want to have a home exercise program. It may seem like too many things to put into practice but proper planning and a good execution will yield great results in the end.

## WAND CLIPS ARE AN INEXPENSIVE WAY TO TRACK YOUR EXERCISES.

A recent study found that holding a wand on your arm during arm curls helped increase the weight lifted by almost 40 percent, compared to doing the same exercise without a wand.

The study shows that the wand clips are easy to use and require minimal equipment and is inexpensive to buy. Before using a wand clip, make sure you read all the safety precautions and instructions.

Wand clips are an effective way to perform exercises at home. They are compact, portable and are easy to use. For those looking for a low cost way to get fit, they make a solid investment. You can use them alone, or combine them with other equipment to challenge yourself. Because this are used to hold weight without having to choose between going light or going heavy. The clips are also able to work either arms or legs and the other options work well with many of the common exercises.

If you're looking to start exercising at home, but don't want to shell out for a bunch of equipment, consider strapping on a sports bra and investing in some wand clips. The clips let you hold exercise equipment on your arms and support yourself as you exercise. They are helpful for people with reduced arm strength, limited upper body mobility, flat chested women, and people who want to challenge themselves but are not physically able to perform more difficult exercises.

The wand clips can also be used for exercises that require upper body strength like bicep curls, barbell rows, triceps' extensions and deadlifts. They allow you to easily add resistance by using small hand weights, which come in different colors and shapes depending on your preferences. The clips also work well for core workouts such as sit-ups, crunches and side planks because they require your abdominal muscles to stabilize you when you lift the weight.

## HOW TO KEEP TRACK OF ALL YOUR HOME EXERCISES AND TRACK YOUR PROGRESS?

Keep tracking your progress can help you keep up the momentum and avoid falling right back into your old habits. So many people start a new exercise, but then never stick with it because they are did not keep track of their progress. How to keep track of your progress?

**These are some ways to keep track of your progress:**

- Create a chart. Some people like to use a calendar, so they can mark off each week as they progress. Others like the look of a chart where they can track their progress month by month. Either way, it is up to you how you choose to mark off your exercise periods so be creative and find something that works for you!
- Use a fitness app or fitness tracker to track your workouts. Many of these apps have special exercise sections where you can track the different exercises and reps for each. Some also have a schedule so you can follow along with a routine.
- Keep a log of your home exercises. For example, write down each meal with what type of exercise or activity you did afterward, like how much time you spent on the treadmill or

walking, and any other notes that you might include such as "Woke up early this morning so I decided to do 30 push-ups," etc.

- Write down how you are feeling. This might be a good idea to do at the end of each week or month, when you are tracking your progress. Write down how you felt at the end of each workout and how motivated or energized you felt.

- Make sure to notice any changes in your weight over time. For instance weight loss or gain. - Maintain a food log and activity tracker to monitor your diet and exercise. This is a good way to keep track of your calories and activity, which will help you make sure that you are getting everything that you need to stay healthy. You can find tons of free apps online to start tracking your activity, food intake, and weight.

- Use a calendar to plan out your workouts for the week and note the date on which they start in your log. You can make a weekly schedule and add in a lot of variety to your workouts. If you have a busy schedule, this can help you keep track of your progress while fitting in things like work and other activities, while still making sure that you are getting the right amount of exercise.

# HOW TO KEEP STAYING MOTIVATED WITH YOUR HOME EXERCISES

## HOW TO KEEP MOTIVATED WITH YOUR HOME EXERCISES AFTER THE FIRST FEW WEEKS OR MONTHS.

It certainly gets easier for many people to stick to their fitness goals as time goes on - it definitely does not get easy, but things get a bit more manageable. Many people find that they have one or two days where they don't do anything at all, and these days are where the real trouble starts. It's important to remember that you got out of the most difficult times by sticking with your routine and adjusting your habits toward a healthier lifestyle. So if you have missed your goal for a few days, make sure to get back on track as soon as possible.

Remember that it may takes 21 days to form a habit - if you miss a day or two, don't give up. Get back to your usual routine quickly and within three weeks you will be back into your routine. A study done in the 60s showed that it takes about 21 days of repetition for someone to form an exercise habit. It takes about half as long for someone to form a bad routine. It's worth it to keep at it!

*To keep you motivated and avoid injury these are few things that you can do:*

- Increase your rest periods if they seem to get a bit too boring. Tire yourself out hard, then take a break. Don't push yourself too hard though. Resting is an important part of exercise and recovery - the harder you work during your rest period, the more you will benefit from that workout session.
- Make sure you do something fun with your exercise. Find a friend or partner to exercise with, or play a game. This could make the time go by faster and allow you to focus on the positive rather than feeling stressed and bored. Try different kinds of exercise - it's always good to mix it up a bit, so don't feel like you have to stick with one type of workout over and over again.
- Engage in some relaxation beforehand and after your workout. Make sure you are physically and mentally relaxed before starting, and make sure you wind down after stopping. When you are in a good mood, you will be more likely to enjoy your workout.
- Don't forget about the basic needs of your body - get enough sleep, enough water, and make sure that you're getting enough food. If you're hungry or tired, it's going to be hard to exercise. Make sure you're comfortable during your workouts. Make sure you feel strong doing the exercises - if you're feeling weak or exhausted, you might need to back off a little bit. You should feel like you're challenged, but not like you want to quit because of the difficulty of the exercise.
- Keep moving, even if you're not doing as much as you'd like to. Take the stairs instead of the elevator. Stand up when you're talking on the phone or watching TV. Stay active and healthy, and it will come naturally to maintain a fitness routine.
- Don't forget that any exercise is better than no exercise at all. Even if it's hard for you to get going, do a little bit - even just a 5 minute calisthenic routine can be beneficial.

- Don't be afraid of failure. Success will come when you're patient and work hard - the road to success is paved with a lot of failures. It's important to keep trying as long as you're having fun, even if it doesn't seem like much is happening. You'll find that your endurance and strength will increase over time, and that new little tricks will start to become second nature.

## 6 WARNINGS ABOUT HOW LONG IT WILL TAKE YOU TO SEE RESULTS FROM HOME EXERCISES.

Exercising from home is a good way to save time and money. But not everyone has the motivation or energy to keep it up when they start making excuses for skipping workouts or slacking off on diets. But more importantly, because of the limited equipment available at home, you may be tempted to compensate by overcompensating or overdoing it. In other words, you may try to work out too hard or do too many reps or sets.

This can lead to injuries that keep you from exercising for weeks or months. Here are 6 warnings about how long it will take you to see results from home exercises.

### 1. You will see results from home exercises much sooner than you realize.

People who exercise at home typically do it for shorter periods, which means that they need to work out longer to see results. The most important thing is to be consistent. Just like with working out in the gym, the body will not respond the same way when muscles are exercised at home. That's why people with experience need a bit more time to see these results, but there is no doubt that they are real and are progress, not just "exercising harder".

## 2. Count on it taking more time to see the results you want.

This is one of the toughest things to deal with because people want results now. You can't just snap your fingers and expect to drop the weight as fast as you want, especially if you're overweight or out of shape.

## 3. Be prepared to feel tired and sore at first, especially if you have not been exercising regularly.

If you have never exercised before, or if it has been a long time since you've worked out, your body takes a little while to get used to it. The muscles are not accustomed to the stress and strain, and therefore it can be quite painful. The very important thing is that you don't give up because it will get better. It will take time, just like you would expect if you were to start exercising in a gym.

## 4. Remember that losing weight does not happen overnight or even within a week or two.

It usually takes weeks of exercise in combination with healthy eating for you to see changes in your body, especially if your goal is to lose weight.

## 5. Know that it will take time to get rid of all the fat you want to lose.

For example, if you are working on building your legs and thighs, it may seem as though there is no change in size at all, but over time, your legs will be stronger and your thighs will be firmer. Sometimes the gains you see in muscle are not obvious until several weeks later.

## 6. Expect to get stronger with home exercises.

Your muscles get stronger by training them. But home exercises are not the same as working out in a gym, so you may need to build up your muscles gradually for these exercises to be more effective at helping you build muscle and burn fat at the same time.

The length time for you to see the progress is not only dependent on your fitness level, but also on the exercises you do. The faster you want results, the longer it will take you to see them. If you are in good shape and have a high fitness level, then it may take only a few weeks to start seeing results. If you are overweight or an out of shape, then it will probably be longer before you see results.

Please don't give up in the early stages and keep going because you'll see changes happen over time and that's just how things go.

## HOW TO STAY MOTIVATED WITH YOUR HOME EXERCISES FOR LONG-TERM RESULTS.

Motivation is important if you want to get fit. The whole point of wanting to get more active is so you can feel healthier, look better, and live a longer life. If you want to motivate yourself, then do something that will be a great achievement. If you want to get fit it is important that you enjoy the activities you are doing. Find a way to motivate yourself by not making working out as a chore, but something fun.

Here are some great ways to get motivated:

### Have a goal in mind

To get motivated, set a fitness goal. It really helps to know what you want if you are looking for exercises. Goals should be measurable, attainable and realistic; so seek out something that is challenging but not too difficult for you to accomplish. When you have a goal in mind, it will get you motivated to accomplish your workout plan.

### Get rid of negativity

If you are a negative person, it will be very hard to get motivated. If you tell yourself that you are not going to eat right or put the effort into finding out how to get motivated and get fit, then why would you actually care? If you want to accomplish your goal, try to keep a positive attitude.

It will be a lot easier to get motivated when you don't have any negativity on your mind.

## Start Small

If you feel like you need something more challenging in order to accomplish your goal, pick something that is easier for you to start with. It doesn't matter of how big or small your goal is; just make sure you start small. If you are struggling to get motivated, starting with something smaller will help you to feel better about your accomplishment.

## Be encouraged by others

If you know any friends or family that can help motivate you, ask them to join you in getting fit. Just ask someone to take the time to go for a walk with you or explain how they feel about getting fit. Talking about it and getting support from friends or family is one of the best ways to get motivated.

## Reward yourself

Once you have accomplished your goal, reward yourself. Reward yourself with dinner out or a new pair of shoes. If you want to motivate yourself, give yourself something for working out and trying to get fit. The more you reward yourself, the more likely you will keep working out.

## Improve yourself

If you want to motivate others, find something you can do well at. For example, if you are the best ballerina in the class and want to be an athlete, begin by finding something that you can achieve as an athlete. So instead of focusing on what you are horrible at, find out what you are good at. You will be more motivated if you feel like you can achieve your goal because you will have already accomplished a goal before even trying.

These are great ways to get motivated for working out. You do not have to be a gym rat or a professional athlete in order to get motivated. You just need to find something that helps you feel like you can accomplish what you want.

13

THE TOP 10 MISTAKES PEOPLE
MAKING WHEN IMPLEMENTING
HOME EXERCISES

Mistakes are common in implementing home exercises. They can be caused by a lack of knowledge or because the person does not know how to adapt to the exercises.

*Here are the top 10 mistakes people make when implementing home exercises:*

**Mistake number one:** *Not knowing what you are doing.* People think that they know what to do but in reality, they do not. They just follow the instructions and try to perform the exercise as it is explained.

The first thing that happens in this case is that the person starts to exercise the wrong muscles, which leads to injury. The person has to take the time to know what muscle he or she is performing a strength exercise for and which muscle group can be targeted in an exercise.

**Mistake number two:** *Being careless.* This is the result of not knowing what you are doing. People do not care about their posture while exercising, they exercise without purpose or aim and in general do not follow instructions. This leads to a lack of results and adverse effects on the body and even greater problems for the person's health.

In this case, the person lacks knowledge and does not know what muscle group is being targeted. They do not care about their posture while exercising, they exercise without purpose or aim and in general do not follow instructions. This leads to a lack of results and adverse effects on the body and even greater problems for the person's health.

**Mistake number three:** *Lacking motivation.* As a result of mistakes one and two, people lose motivation to continue exercising at home. They can never imagine the results that they see at the gym so they decide to stop.

**Mistake number four:** *Trying to do everything by yourself.* People think that home exercises require only physical exercise and they do not involve other areas of the body such as muscles, bones, ligaments, etc. This is a mistake because it does not consider all the useful characteristics of home exercises. There are many benefits from home exercises besides just being able to build muscles and tone your body.

**Mistake number five:** *Trying to do too many exercises at the same time.* This happens when people see a lot of good and different exercises for home training. They try doing all of them at the same time and lose track of what they are doing. Then they start doing the wrong exercises and this leads to injury or symptoms of low body function.

**Mistake number six:** *Not exercising very often enough.* People think that they have to exercise daily in order to get results. In reality, there is no need to exercise daily; just a few times a week will suffice because home exercises require time, motivation, and hard work. Do not feel bad if you miss a day of exercising; it happens to everyone and the only thing you have to do is continue with the practice.

**Mistake number seven:** *Lacking patience.* People try many new things at the same time and expect great results just after one or two weeks of training. This is a mistake and the main reason why most people quit exercising at home. The body needs time to adapt to the exercises and in order to obtain results, you have to be patient.

**Mistake number eight:** *Not having respect for your body and health.* This is a usual mistake and the main reason why many people lose motivation to exercise at home. People think that they are not working hard enough in order to obtain results. They believe that exercises are not a good thing because they do more harm than good.

**Mistake number nine:** *Ignoring the feeling of failure.* When a person does not know what they are doing, they do not feel the results and therefore do not give enough importance to achieving them.

In this case, the person does not give importance to feeling the stretch or the burning sensation in their muscles. They also ignore how their body reacts at the end of an exercise because they have not felt any change and therefore give no value to it.

**Mistake number ten:** *Over-training.* This happens when people train too often and do not recover enough between workouts. This leads to fatigue and the risk of overuse injuries.

In this case, the person does not respect what their body tells them and does not listen to it. If their body feels like resting for a day or two then they should rest; otherwise, they risk overtraining.

As you can see from these mistakes, there are many things that people should know in order to implement a home exercise program properly. As you now know, home exercises require time, effort, and hard work. They are not a miracle that you have to perform just for the sake of it. If you do them correctly and with patience, it will lead to very positive results.

14

# TIPS FOR A SUCCESSFUL HOME EXERCISE PROGRAM

## 6 TIPS FOR A SUCCESSFUL HOME EXERCISE PROGRAM IN YOUR HOME.

To be successful with your fitness program, you need to understand your own body and personal motivation. Some people are motivated by the way that physical activity makes them feel, while others will only exercise if they have a specific goal in mind before they begin. You might need to experiment with different types of exercise and fitness activities to determine what it is that will motivate you to stay active.

Some tips to keep your motivation high and help you get fit at home:

### 1. Take it easy on yourself

You don't need to push yourself beyond your limit. On the contrary, you should take things easy and give your body time to adjust. You can gradually increase the intensity of your workouts or add new exercises as you feel ready for them.

## 2. Make sure the exercises are working

Once you've become comfortable with an exercise, make sure it's still effective. Don't be afraid to change things if you aren't getting results or if you're tired of doing them every day. Doing a few pushups every day won't build you the arms of an Olympic sprinter. You'll have to switch things up if you want to see significant results.

## 3. Be consistent

Try to avoid being inconsistent with your workouts because this will weaken your body and make it harder for you to work out when you get back into the habit again. Make a commitment and stick to it.

## 4. Don't buy into the hype

You don't need fancy workout machines or a huge DVD collection. Just focus on doing the basic exercises and you'll be fine.

## 5. Be honest with yourself

Don't beat yourself over the head for not working out enough or not being able to lift as much weight as your workout partner. Remember that at-home workouts are just as effective as those in a gym, and it's not about who does more pushups or runs faster on the treadmill. If you're using the right techniques, both of these things will work.

## 6. Take the time to enjoy your workouts

By focusing on what you're doing, you'll be more likely to do it because you'll have fun and enjoy it. It's about developing a habit to do something that is beneficial for your body. And by doing so at home, it can become a part of your daily routine, which will keep you motivated all the time!

## A SMALL YARD WORK CAN GO A LONG WAY

If you're like most people, you don't have a ton of time to spend at the gym every day. But that doesn't mean you can't stay in shape! There are some easy and efficient home exercises that can get your heart rate up in just minutes just like a little yard work.

A small yard work can go a long way if you're looking for a quick workout that won't break the bank. These home exercises can be done anywhere, anytime and require nothing more than a good pair of shoes, some elbow grease, and the willingness to give everything you've got. The following is a list of great exercises you can do in your yard:

Give yourself four minutes to complete each exercise and one minute rest between each exercise. After you complete all exercises, give yourself ten minutes of rest and then repeat the entire workout again. This will get you a total of 40 home exercises in a twenty minute period.

The bottom line is that getting your heart rate up at home doesn't have to be complicated. Try this workout and you'll be surprised at how much better you feel after just one time around!

## Garden Hose Walk

1. Find a hula hoop, garden hose, or anything similar to use as your track.
2. Walk in a line with your hula hoop or garden hose in front of you.
3. Perform the exercise for 10-20 steps before walking backward for 10-20 steps, slowly turning the hose as you turn.
4. Repeat this exercise for approximately 20 minutes, gradually increasing time as your fitness level improves over a period of time.

## Leg Press

1. Find a small step ladder.
2. Take one foot off the ground and push up on your toes without bending your knees.

3. Slowly lower yourself to the ground and repeat this exercise with your other foot.
4. Continue this cycle for 20 minutes, for a total of 40 repetitions.

## Mow the Lawn

1. Find a small piece of yard to mow; it doesn't have to be huge.
2. Mow the lawn by walking behind the lawn mower without pushing it. (This will give you hand and arm work as well as leg work.
3. Never push the mower, you're only using your legs.
4. Continue to mow the lawn for 20 minutes for a total of 40 repetitions.

## Digging Out

1. Use a shovel to dig away dirt from any area in your yard.
2. Make sure the hole is deep enough and wide enough to make digging uncomfortable. (This exercise requires you to forcefully push up on the shovel with each step, so be prepared).
3. Continue digging for 20 minutes for a total of 40 repetitions.

## Plant Flower Beds

1. Dig up the flower beds in your yard.
2. Plant three to five different kinds of flowers in the holes you dig.
3. Once the flower bed is about an inch deep, replace the soil on top of each bed.
4. Water each bed thoroughly.
5. Continue this exercise for 20 minutes, for a total of 40 repetitions.

## Hauling Compost

1. Find a wheelbarrow and fill it with a combination of grass clippings, soil and leaves.
2. Roll the wheelbarrow for 20 minutes.
3. This exercise will require you to move your arms, shoulders, back and legs in order to complete 40 repetitions.

## Pulling Weeds

1. Dig into the soil with your garden weeder and pull up any weeds you see.
2. Continue this workout for 20 minutes for a total of 40 repetitions.

## Trimming the Grass

1. Use an edger to cut the grass in your yard.
2. Cut 15 inches at a time and then switch to the other side and cut 15 inches at a time.
3. Repeat this exercise for 20 minutes, for a total of 40 repetitions.

If you're doing a little yard work each week and work in some of these easy home exercises from time to time, you'll have the best of both worlds: fit body and a nice yard! So go out there and get your yard work on! The best part is that a little yard work can go a long way!

## ESTABLISH A HEALTHY DAILY ROUTINE?

Routines are essential for us to function as human beings, allowing us to remember the numerous processes we have to go through in our lives. Establishing a routine helps us to create an order in our day, and it trains the brain to manage attention.

Routines help us to manage our time efficiently and make sure we're getting the most out of it. For exercise, it seems that defining a routine may seem like an intimidating task, however, when we make a plan for exercise in terms of timing and frequency, we can actually make it more accessible than initially expected. It can help combat the sense of confinement on our bodies that come with being sedentary. We all know that being physically active and fit is important to our health and well-being.

Create a routine. We all have one, it's just that we don't always use it. The following are some basic exercises that should be incorporated into your "dance card" or exercise plan so you can have a new and exciting routine to keep you fit at home without leaving the comfort of your own home.

You can exercise for three days a week and rotate your routines. For example, if you exercise on Monday, Wednesday and Friday, your routine can be:

**MONDAY:** Stair aerobics,

**WEDNESDAY:** Chair aerobics with weights

**FRIDAY:** Weight training in your home.

**Wednesday (after work):** Yoga.

One of the best ways of adding activity into your day is by combining walking with other tasks. You can read while exercising by holding a book and taking long steps. You can also make up phone calls or do paperwork while exercising even if you don't have an office. Even activities such as vacuuming and sweeping the floor are great ways to add activity into your day.

It is essential to create small achievable goals for yourself. It is important that you set attainable goals for yourself that are realistic. Don't overwork yourself by attempting to achieve too many goals at once, instead, take it one step at a time and achieve them.

If there's a great thing we have learned, it's how to turn a habit into an enjoyable routine. We all have different ways of achieving a common goal. Take the time to think about the things you enjoy doing and try to incorporate those activities into your daily routine. If you like a challenge, take up new challenges as challenges tend to breed success and can also provide extra motivation for you. Many people are now realizing the importance of physical activity in their lives and are incorporating it into their daily routine. Find what works for you and make a plan that fits your schedule. You'll be surprised how easy exercises can be when you set yourself up for success in a routine that fits your lifestyle.

Posture work is as important as strength training in building strength and muscle mass. It is an essential part of a healthy lifestyle, no matter what kind of workout routines are outside the home. When it comes to posture, it might not be as noticeable, and yet, it can be just as important as strength training for maintaining good posture, and giving yourself the best chance of avoiding back pain.

It is vital to find a way to ensure that you don't lose your back strength and flexibility. In order for this to happen, you'll need to work both your upper and lower body simultaneously in one exercise session. The best way to do this is combining both forms of exercise into one routine.

Back workouts are quite simple and easy to do, as long as you have a few basic tools in your home, such as:

- Backpack straps or resistance bands
- Rubber exercise balls
- Medicine balls

These tools can help you to perform the exercises in this workout routine at a high intensity that will build up your strength and flexibility.

# 15

# QUOTES ON HOW TO INCREASE STRENGTH / MUSCLE MASS

Getting into shape is no easy task, and weight-training is not always an option. If you have a limited amount of time to exercise and don't want to spend money on expensive machines, it can be very hard to find the time. Despite these difficulties, there are still ways you can exercise at home without even leaving your house! Below are 10 quotes on how to increase strength, increase muscle mass, and stay in shape without ever leaving your living room!

**1. "Success is not final, failure is not fatal: it is the courage to continue that counts." – Winston Churchill**

- The quote above is a great way to wake yourself up in the morning and get your motivation going. Having a strong will helps you persevere in the face of failure, which will help you stay consistent with training.

**2. "If you don't stand up for something, you'll fall for anything." – Maya Angelou**

- The quote above is a great way to make sure you're pushing yourself hard and consistently by considering how you will know when it's time to stop.

*3. "You can do anything you set your mind to. The decision to succeed or fail, to be rich or poor, great or small depends on that single thoughtless act of pursuit or acceptance." – Jay Zawodney*

- This quote is a good reminder to not be afraid to work hard. Your level of success is entirely up to you as long as you're willing to put in the work!

*4. "There are no rules in the NFL, and if there were, the Bucs would have invented them." - Dan Marino*

- Although this quote isn't directly about training for weight-loss, it could apply very well during your journey.

*5. "To build a dream, you must wake up." —Roald Dahl*

- Waking yourself up out of a daydream can be difficult, but it's necessary. Training yourself out of laziness is important when trying to find the motivation to stay fit.

*6. "A person is punished in this life more by what he does not do than by what he does do." —Albert Einstein*

- Although this quote isn't directly about weight-loss, it's a good reminder when you're trying to find a balance between what you do and what you don't do.

*7. "Whatever you do, make sure it is the right thing at the right time. This is more important than anything else." —Johann Wolfgang Von Goethe*

- This quote is great for helping you realize what needs to be done. Don't rush past the small things and make sure you do the important things when they need to be done!

**8. "It begins by taking small steps. It's not a sprint, it's a marathon. So keep moving and don't stop until you get to where you want to be." —Njeri Wanyeki**

- This quote is a great way to remind yourself that results are slow and can take a while. Train consistently at first, but don't get discouraged if your progress is slow after a couple of weeks.

**9. "It's hard to beat a person who never gives up." – Babe Ruth**

- Never giving up is very important when it comes to weight-loss and staying in shape. Make sure you have an attitude that will help you stay with it and not give up!

**10. "If you tell the truth, you don't have to remember anything." – Mark Twain**

- Weight-loss is all about being honest with yourself. If your diet or exercise plan isn't working out, tell yourself and fix it!

**11. "It's easier to go up the stairs than to stop going down."**

- A great quote on exercising! If you want to exercise, you have to keep doing it. Even if it's a struggle, just keep at it until you reach your goal.

**12. "You can accomplish anything you want if your mind is in the right place and if your heart is in God's hands." —Malcolm X**

- This quote about weight-loss is a great reminder to always have a positive attitude and be sure that you're doing it for yourself.

**13. "If you don't take action, you won't make any money. If you keep failing, don't give up on yourself, quit and get a better job." —Bill Gate**

- This quote is great for reminding yourself to not be lazy and take action when you have a chance.

**14. "No one can make you feel inferior without your consent." —
Eleanor Roosevelt**

- This quote about weight-loss is a great reminder that everyone has every right to feel good about themselves, and that it's important not to let others make you feel bad about yourself.

**15. "You're going to fail. That's a given. You're going to fail often. But you're not going to be able to fail if you don't try something."**

- Andrew Carnegie said that. He was extremely rich and he kept on doing what made him feel good even when everyone was against him! The quote really proves that if you keep moving forward, things will go your way eventually. And always remember, "You can do anything you set your mind to."

These quotes list should help motivate you when it comes to training at home. If you're trying to lose weight or build muscle, I hope that these quotes helped you on your journey!

# CONCLUSION

Exercises are at the same time a very popular and a very old method of training the muscles. Today there are various kinds of exercises that can be done at home, by one person or with several participants for professional purposes or as a hobby.

Home exercises are one of the best things you can do to feel good about yourself and incorporate exercise into your daily routine.

Today many people are busier than ever and often find it difficult to find time for exercise. For many, they can't even figure out where to begin with all the choices available today. For those who don't have access to a gym or fitness center within their own home, there are still ways that you can get in shape without a workout at your local health club.

You can start by doing some simple stretching exercises to help get your ready for your workout. The next thing that you should do is try and increase the intensity of your workout, so that you're building muscle while still burning lots of calories. There are several different home exercise routines that you can follow on your own, or with your family.

For instance, the first thing in the morning, you can have your kids do some jumping jacks while you stretch to get limber and warm up. Then as soon as you're ready to start working out, have them do some jumping jacks while you use some free weights to complete a circuit of muscle-building exercises.

There's a lot of benefits to working out at home. For one thing, it's less expensive than going to a gym and for those on a budget, that's an added benefit. But for people who are really busy, working out at home provides the encouragement that they need to get in shape.

You can pick up some free weights and dumbbells at your local home improvement store and use them to work out on your own. You can get some exercise with your children or grandchildren as well. This can be a great bonding experience for you and your family.

There are many kinds of home exercises that you can do as part of your daily regimen. The more exercise you get, the better shape you'll be in, and the easier it will be to get back into the routine again if you have to miss a week or two for whatever reason.

Always remember that working out has a lot of benefits for your overall health and well-being. It's a great way to stay on track with your diet, and it's an excellent way to lose weight even when you're not dieting. Consistency is what you need to accomplish your goals, so be sure to get your workouts in, and in the end, you'll feel better about yourself.

I hope you got some knowledge from this book to be more happy and healthy.

# REFERENCES

Angelini, M., n.d. Aerobic responses to 12 weeks of training on various modes of home exercise equipment in sedentary adults.

BrainyQuote. 2021. Success Quotes - BrainyQuote. [Online] Available at: <https://www.brainyquote.com/topics/success-quotes> [Accessed 10 July 2021].

GearHungry. 2021. Best Gym Equipment for Your Home - Gear Hungry. [online] Available at: <https://www.gearhungry.com/best-home-gym-equipment/> [Accessed 10 July 2021].

Good Housekeeping. 2021. 15 Easy Workout Moves You Can Do at Home. [online] Available at: <https://www.goodhousekeeping.com/health/fitness/a31478709/home-workout/> [Accessed 10 July 2021].

GymPerson.com. 2021. How to Stay Motivated to Workout at Home – 10 Tips. [online] Available at: <https://gymperson.com/home-workout-motivation/> [Accessed 10 July 2021].

Healthline. 2020. 10 Best Exercises for Everyone. [online] Available at: <https://www.healthline.com/health/fitness-exercise/10-best-exercises-everyday> [Accessed 10 July 2021].

Nerd Fitness. 2021. Bodyweight Workout for Beginners: 20-Minute at Home Routine | Nerd Fitness. [online] Available at: <https://www.nerd-fitness.com/blog/beginner-body-weight-workout-burn-fat-build-muscle> [Accessed 10 July 2021].

Schaefer, A., 2010. Exercise. Chicago, Ill.: Heinemann Library.